Community Pharmacy: A Practical Approach

EMAD SALEM

Copyright © 2024 Emad Salem

All rights reserved.

ISBN: 979-8-3408-3601-4

INTRODUCTION

Community pharmacy plays a vital role in the healthcare system, serving as the most accessible point of care for many patients. Pharmacists are not only responsible for dispensing medications but also for providing essential health advice, managing minor ailments, and supporting patients in their overall healthcare journey. The role of the community pharmacist has evolved significantly, with an increased focus on patient-centered care, health education, and disease prevention.

This book, Community Pharmacy: A Practical Approach, is designed to serve as a comprehensive guide for pharmacy students, recent graduates, and early-career pharmacists. It aims to bridge the gap between academic learning and real-world practice, providing practical insights into the day-to-day responsibilities of a community pharmacist. The information is organized to offer clear, actionable advice on managing common health conditions, counseling patients, and making informed recommendations on over-the-counter (OTC) treatments.

Purpose of the Book

The primary goal of this book is to empower pharmacists with the knowledge and skills needed to provide high-quality patient care in a community setting. Whether you are a pharmacy student looking to build a solid foundation or a new graduate navigating the complexities of patient interactions, this guide offers practical tools and strategies for success.

Importance of Community Pharmacy

As frontline healthcare providers, community pharmacists often serve as the first point of contact for patients seeking medical advice. In many cases, patients visit their local pharmacist before consulting with a physician. This places a significant responsibility on pharmacists to offer accurate, timely, and empathetic care.

Beyond dispensing medications, pharmacists play a crucial role in ensuring medication safety, educating patients about their treatments, and promoting public health initiatives such as vaccinations and chronic disease management. This book highlights the pharmacist's multifaceted role and the growing importance of community pharmacy in delivering comprehensive healthcare.

What to Expect from this Book

The chapters in this book are organized to cover key areas of community pharmacy practice:

1. **Effective Communication:** The first chapter explores the importance of building strong relationships with patients through active listening, empathy, and clear communication.
2. **Managing Common Conditions:** Subsequent chapters provide practical guidance on treating common respiratory, digestive, skin, and eye conditions. You'll learn how to assess symptoms, make OTC recommendations, and identify when to refer patients for further medical care.
3. **Specialized Care:** Dedicated chapters focus on pediatric and women's health, offering insights into managing conditions unique to these populations.
4. **Patient-Centered Counseling:** Each chapter emphasizes the importance of patient education, empowering pharmacists to provide thorough and personalized health advice.
5. **Practical Tools and Case Studies:** Throughout the book, you will find real-world case studies, practical tips, and common patient questions to enhance your understanding of pharmacy practice.

This book is intended to serve as both a learning tool and a day-to-day reference guide. It has been carefully structured to offer clear, concise, and practical advice, while also emphasizing the ethical and professional responsibilities of pharmacists in providing patient-centered care.

Final Thoughts

Pharmacy is a constantly evolving profession, and the knowledge shared in this book reflects the latest practices in community pharmacy. However, healthcare is always advancing, and it is essential to stay updated on new guidelines, treatments, and best practices. As you read through this book, I hope it enhances your skills, sharpens your understanding of pharmacy practice, and prepares you to meet the needs of the patients you will serve.

Best wishes for your journey into community pharmacy,
Dr. Emad Salem

NOTE

I would like to express my deepest gratitude to everyone who contributed to the successful completion of this book. Special thanks go to my colleagues, friends, and family for their unwavering support throughout the writing process. I am also thankful to the review and editing teams for their invaluable input, guidance, and feedback.

Community Pharmacy: A Practical Approach aims to provide a comprehensive, practical guide for pharmacy students, recent graduates, and early-career pharmacists. The information contained within this book has been thoroughly researched and presented with the intention of supporting the development of essential skills that enable pharmacists to deliver high-quality patient care in a community setting.

Despite the extensive efforts put into ensuring the accuracy and reliability of the information in this book, pharmacy is a dynamic and rapidly evolving field. Guidelines, treatments, and best practices continue to change, so readers are encouraged to stay updated with the latest developments in the profession through continuous learning and reference to the most current guidelines.

I sincerely hope that this book serves as a valuable resource, enhancing your knowledge, refining your skills, and contributing to your growth as a pharmacist. Your feedback, suggestions, and insights are always welcome as they will help improve future editions of this work.

Thank you, and I wish you success in your career as a pharmacist.

Best wishes,
Dr. Emad Salem

CONTENTS

Chapter 1: Communication with Patients.	1	**Chapter 6: Minor eye Conditions**	111
Chapter 2: Respiratory Conditions	14	Part 1: Conjunctivitis	115
Part 1: Cough	15	Part 2: Dry eye syndrome	117
Part 2: Common Cold	20	Part 3: Blepharitis	119
Chapter 3: Gastrointestinal Health	33	**Chapter 7: Women's health**	125
Part 1: Constipation	35	Part 1: Menstrual disorders	127
Part 2: Diarrhea	43	Part 2: UTI	129
Part 3: IBS	49	Part 3: Menopause	131
Part 4: GERD	56	Part 4: Osteoporosis	133
Chapter 4: Skin conditions	71	**Chapter 8: Neurological Conditions**	138
Part 1: Hair loss	74	Part 1: Insomnia	139
Part 2: Cold sores	76	Part 2: Motion Sickness	144
Part 3: Athlete's foot	79		
Part 4: Dandruff	82		
Part 5: Eczema	85		
Part 6: Warts	88		
Part 7: Scabies	91		
Chapter 5: Pediatric Health	100		
Part 1: Oral thrush	102		
Part 2: Colic	104		
Part 3: Pinworm	106		
Part 4: Napkin rash	108		

CHAPTER 1: COMMUNICATION WITH PATIENTS.

I. Introduction
Role of the Pharmacist in Patient Communication

1. **Medication Guidance**: Pharmacists explain the purpose of medications, how they work, correct dosage, potential side effects, and interactions. They ensure patients understand their medication regimen.
2. **Health Counseling**: They provide advice on lifestyle changes, diet, exercise, and self-care to manage health conditions. They also counsel on preventive care like vaccinations.
3. **Patient Education**: Pharmacists educate patients about their health conditions, helping them understand the importance of adhering to their treatment plans.
4. **Empathy and Support**: Pharmacists provide emotional support, especially when patients are dealing with challenging health issues. They must show understanding, patience, and empathy.
5. **Advocacy**: They advocate for patients, particularly in issues related to medication costs, insurance, and accessibility to healthcare services.
6. **Collaboration**: Pharmacists collaborate with other healthcare professionals, participating in shared decision-making processes to provide coordinated care to the patient.

7. **Crisis Management**: In times of health crises or emergencies, pharmacists play a crucial role in providing accurate information, dispelling myths, and guiding patients.
8. **Confidentiality**: They maintain the privacy and confidentiality of patient information, a vital aspect of professional ethics and patient rights.

II. Basic Communication Skills
A. Active Listening

Active listening is fully focusing on, understanding, and responding to a speaker, and remembering what the speaker has said. It fosters understanding, builds rapport, and encourages patients to share more about their health issues, leading to more effective patient care.

Techniques:

1. **Eye contact**: Shows you're focused and interested in what the patient is saying.
2. **Nodding**: Non-verbal acknowledgment shows you're following along.
3. **Paraphrasing**: Restating the speaker's words in your own words to confirm understanding.
4. **Reflecting**: Reflecting back feelings and emotions can show empathy and understanding.
5. **Clarifying questions**: Asking questions to ensure understanding or to get more information.
6. **Summarizing**: Summarizing the main points can help ensure you and the patient are on the same page.
7. **Barriers**: Identify common barriers to active listening, such as distractions, preconceived notions, or language differences, and discuss how to overcome them.

B. Empathy and Respect

Empathy is the ability to understand and share the feelings of others, while respect is acknowledging the value and worth of individuals and treating them with dignity. Empathy and respect are fundamental to building a positive and trusting relationship with patients. They help patients feel valued, understood, and more comfortable discussing their health concerns.

Techniques:

1. **Use supportive language**: The language should be non-judgmental and sensitive to the patient's feelings and experiences.
2. **Active listening**: This shows you genuinely care about their concerns.
3. **Show understanding**: Express understanding of the patient's feelings and concerns. This could be as simple as saying, *"I can see why you'd feel that way."*
4. **Maintain eye contact**: This can convey respect and that you're fully engaged in the conversation.
5. **Validate feelings**: Acknowledge the patient's emotions and reassure them that their feelings are valid.
6. **Respect for diversity**: Discuss the importance of respecting patients' cultural, social, and personal values.

C. Verbal and Non-verbal Communication

Verbal communication involves the use of words to convey messages, while non-verbal communication involves actions, gestures, facial expressions, body language, tone of voice, and other visual cues. Both verbal and non-verbal communication play crucial roles in conveying information, showing empathy, building trust, and understanding the patient's emotions and concerns.

Verbal Communication Techniques:

1. **Clarity**: Use simple, clear, and straightforward language.
2. **Tone**: The tone of voice should be calm, friendly, and respectful.
3. **Pace**: Speak at a moderate pace to ensure understanding.
4. **Confirmation**: Regularly confirm if the patient understands the information.

Non-verbal Communication Techniques:

1. **Body Language**: Maintain an open posture, and avoid crossing arms or legs, which can seem defensive.
2. **Eye Contact**: Demonstrates engagement and sincerity.
3. **Facial Expressions**: Should be consistent with the message being conveyed.
4. **Gestures**: Use appropriate hand and arm movements to enhance verbal communication.
5. **Physical Distance**: Respect personal space to avoid making the patient uncomfortable.

6. **Interpreting Non-verbal cues**: Discuss the importance of observing and accurately interpreting the non-verbal cues from patients, such as facial expressions and body language, to understand their feelings and concerns better.

D. Asking the Right Questions

This involves asking specific, open-ended, and closed-ended questions to gather necessary information from patients. It aids in understanding the patient's condition, concerns, and treatment history. It helps in making informed decisions about their healthcare.

Techniques:

1. **Open-ended questions**: These questions encourage patients to share more information. For example, *"Can you describe the pain you're feeling?"*
2. **Closed-ended questions**: These questions are used to get specific information or a 'yes' or 'no' answer. For example, *"Did you take your medicine this morning?"*
3. **Follow-up questions**: These questions are used to clarify or get more detail on a previous response. For example, *"You mentioned a sharp pain in your chest. Can you tell me more about when it happens?"*
4. **Reflective questions**: These questions reflect back what the patient has said, reassuring them that they have been heard and understood. For example, *"It sounds like you're worried about the side effects of this medication, is that correct?"*
5. **Patient-centric Approach**: Questions should be asked with respect and empathy, ensuring the patient feels comfortable and understood.
6. **Privacy and Confidentiality**: Be mindful of the environment when asking sensitive questions. Respect the patient's privacy and confidentiality.

III. Counselling Patients about Medications
A. Explaining Purpose and Benefits of Medication

This involves explaining to the patient why a particular medication has been prescribed, its actions in the body, and the expected benefits. It enhances patient understanding, supports informed decision-making, and improves medication adherence.

Techniques:

1. **Use Simple Language:** Avoid medical jargon and explain in a language that the patient can understand.
2. **Be Specific:** Detail the exact role of the medication in managing the patient's condition.
3. **Discuss Benefits:** Explain the expected benefits, including symptom relief, prevention of disease progression, or cure.
4. **Personalize Information:** Tailor the explanation to the individual patient's condition and context.
5. **Patient Engagement:** Encourage questions and discussions. Ensure the patient understands by asking them to repeat back the information in their own words.
6. **Visual Aids:** Use visual aids where appropriate to help explain complex information.
7. **Privacy and Respect:** Ensure these discussions are held privately and respectfully, considering the patient's comfort and dignity.

B. Discussing Possible Side Effects

This involves informing the patient about potential adverse effects of a medication, their signs and symptoms, and what to do if they occur. It prepares patients for what to expect, helps them identify serious side effects quickly, and helps reduce anxiety and fear associated with unknown outcomes.

Techniques:

1. **Be Honest:** Clearly communicate the potential side effects, but also reassure patients that not everyone experiences them.
2. **Prioritize:** Discuss the most common and serious side effects. Trying to cover all possible side effects may overwhelm the patient.
3. **Provide Guidance:** Explain what to do if they experience a side effect, including when to seek immediate medical attention.
4. **Use Simple Language:** Explain using clear, non-technical language that the patient can understand.
5. **Balance:** While it's important to discuss side effects, also reassure the patient about the benefits of the medication, to avoid non-compliance due to fear of side effects.

6. **Encourage Reporting**: Encourage patients to report any experienced side effects. This not only helps manage their treatment but also contributes to post-market drug safety surveillance.
7. **Privacy and Respect**: Hold these discussions in a private, quiet place and always respect the patient's feelings and reactions.

C. Instruction on Proper Use and Storage

This involves explaining to the patient how to correctly use their medication and how to store it to maintain its efficacy. Proper use and storage of medication are critical for ensuring its effectiveness and preventing potential harm.
Techniques:

1. **Provide Clear Instructions**: Explain how to take the medication (e.g., with meals or on an empty stomach), at what times, and for how long. Also, explain how to use devices if any (like inhalers or insulin pens).
2. **Discuss Storage**: Discuss optimal storage conditions (like room temperature, avoid sunlight, refrigeration if needed) and what to do if a medication is accidentally left out.
3. **Demonstrate**: If possible, show the patient how to take or use the medication.
4. **Write It Down**: Provide written instructions as a reference for the patient.
5. **Address Misconceptions**: Discuss any common misconceptions or myths about medication use and storage.
6. **Encourage Questions**: Make sure the patient feels comfortable asking questions about their medication.
7. **Follow-up**: Plan for a follow-up to check if the patient is using and storing the medication correctly.

D. Importance of Adherence to Medication

Medication adherence refers to whether patients take their medications as prescribed, including timing, dosage, and frequency. Proper adherence is crucial for the effectiveness of the medication. Non-adherence can lead to treatment failure, worsening of the disease, increased healthcare costs, and potentially preventable hospitalizations.
Techniques:

1. **Education**: Ensure patients understand why they need the medication, how it works, and the consequences of non-adherence.
2. **Simplify Regimens**: If possible, recommend simpler medication regimens (like once-daily dosing or combination pills).
3. **Reminders**: Suggest strategies like setting alarms, using pill boxes, or mobile apps to help remember doses.
4. **Address Concerns**: Discuss any fears or concerns the patient might have, like side effects or cost, which could impact adherence.
5. **Barriers to Adherence**: Identify potential barriers to adherence, such as complex regimens, side effects, cost, forgetfulness, or lack of understanding about the need for the medication, and discuss strategies to overcome these.
6. **Regular Monitoring**: Encourage regular follow-up to monitor adherence and address any issues promptly.

IV. Handling Difficult Conversations
A. Dealing with Angry or Upset Patients

This involves managing interactions with patients who may be angry, upset, or frustrated due to various reasons like long wait times, perceived poor service, or misunderstanding about their treatment. Properly managing these situations helps maintain a positive patient-provider relationship, ensure effective communication, and prevent escalation of conflict.

Techniques:

1. **Remain Calm**: Keep your emotions in check, maintaining a calm and composed demeanor.
2. **Active Listening**: Show empathy and understanding. Let the patient express their feelings without interruption.
3. **Don't Take It Personally**: Understand that the patient's anger is likely due to their situation, not you personally.
4. **Apologize and Acknowledge**: If a mistake has been made, acknowledge it and apologize. Even if no mistake was made, you can still apologize for the patient's feelings of frustration.
5. **Find a Solution**: Once the patient has calmed down, work with them to find a solution to their problem or concern.

6. **De-escalation Tactics**: These can include techniques like maintaining a comfortable distance, using a calm tone of voice, and avoiding confrontational body language.
7. **Self-Care**: Caring for oneself after these encounters is important. Discuss strategies for stress management and emotional well-being.

B. Discussing Sensitive Health Issues

This involves discussing health topics that may be uncomfortable, personal, or stigmatized, such as sexual health, mental health, substance use, or end-of-life decisions. Open and respectful conversation about these issues is crucial for comprehensive patient care and to ensure patients receive the necessary support and treatment.

Techniques:

1. **Create a Safe Space**: Make the patient feel comfortable, ensuring privacy and confidentiality.
2. **Use Empathy**: Show understanding and non-judgment, acknowledging the courage it takes to discuss these issues.
3. **Use Appropriate Language**: Use respectful, patient-centered, non-stigmatizing language. For example, using *"people with substance use disorder"* instead of *"addicts"*.
4. **Ask Permission**: Before discussing sensitive issues, ask the patient if they're comfortable discussing them.
5. **Provide Support**: Offer resources for additional support, such as counseling services or support groups.
6. **Cultural Sensitivity**: Be aware of cultural beliefs and practices that may influence how patients perceive and discuss sensitive health issues.
7. **Legal and Ethical Considerations**: Be aware of laws regarding reporting obligations for certain sensitive issues, like child abuse or threats of harm to self or others.

C. Communicating with Patients with Low Health Literacy

Health literacy is the degree to which individuals can obtain, process, and understand basic health information and services needed to make appropriate health decisions. Patients with low health literacy may struggle to understand medical instructions, make informed health decisions, and manage their health. Effective communication is critical to ensuring they receive appropriate care.

Techniques:

1. **Use Simple Language**: Avoid medical jargon and technical terms. Use plain, everyday language whenever possible.
2. **Use Visual Aids**: Diagrams, models, and other visual aids can help patients understand complex information.
3. **Teach-Back Method**: After explaining a health issue or instruction, ask the patient to repeat back the information in their own words to confirm understanding.
4. **Be Patient and Encouraging**: Allow patients extra time to process information and make decisions. Encourage questions and active participation in their care.
5. **Provide Written Information**: Give patients written instructions or materials to review at home.
6. **Respect and Empathy**: Always approach patients with low health literacy with respect and empathy. Don't make assumptions about their abilities based on their literacy levels.

D. Breaking Bad News

This involves communicating unfavorable information or prognosis to patients and their families, such as a diagnosis of a serious illness, recurrence of disease, or end-of-life decisions. Breaking bad news is an inevitable part of healthcare. It's crucial to do this in an empathetic and clear manner to minimize patient distress and confusion.

Techniques:

1. **Prepare**: Review all relevant clinical information and plan what you will say.
2. **Set the Stage**: Ensure privacy, minimize interruptions, and sit at the patient's level.
3. **Deliver the News**: Use clear and simple language, avoid jargon, and deliver the news directly but empathetically.
4. **Respond to Patient Emotions**: Allow for silence and emotional reactions, provide support, and reassure the patient you will be there to help them through this.
5. **Plan and Follow-Up**: Discuss next steps, answer questions, and arrange for additional support if needed, such as counseling.

6. **SPIKES Protocol**: This is a six-step protocol for breaking bad news, encompassing: Setting up the interview, assessing the patient's Perception, obtaining the patient's Invitation, giving Knowledge and information to the patient, addressing the patient's Emotions with empathic responses, and Strategizing and Summarizing the discussed information.

Chapter Summary

Effective communication is a cornerstone of pharmacy practice. In this chapter, we explored the critical role of pharmacists in patient communication, including medication guidance, health counseling, and emotional support. Pharmacists must develop active listening skills, empathy, and the ability to respect diverse backgrounds to build trust and rapport with patients.

Key skills covered include:
1. Active Listening: Focusing fully on patients' concerns and responding appropriately to ensure understanding.
2. Empathy and Respect: Demonstrating understanding of patients' feelings and maintaining a respectful, non-judgmental approach.
3. Verbal and Non-Verbal Communication: Using clear language, appropriate tone, and body language to convey information and support.
4. Counseling on Medications: Educating patients on the purpose, benefits, side effects, and proper use of medications to improve adherence and outcomes.
5. Handling Difficult Conversations: Strategies for managing interactions with upset or distressed patients, and discussing sensitive health issues while maintaining professionalism.

Mastering these communication skills enhances the pharmacist's ability to deliver comprehensive healthcare, fostering better patient outcomes and satisfaction.

Practical Activity
Role Play Scenarios (e.g., counselling a patient, dealing with a difficult conversation)

1. Counseling a Patient on a New Medication:

Pharmacist: Explains why the new medication has been prescribed, how to take it, possible side effects, and answers any questions.
Patient: Asks questions about the medication, expresses concerns about side effects and cost.

2. Breaking Bad News:

Doctor: Breaks the news of a cancer diagnosis using the SPIKES protocol.
Patient: Reacts to the news, asks questions about prognosis and treatment options.

3. Dealing with an Angry Patient:

Nurse: Deals with a patient who is upset about waiting too long for their appointment.
Patient: Expresses frustration and anger about the wait time, feels they're not being taken seriously.

4. Discussing Sensitive Health Issues:

Counselor: Discusses a recent diagnosis of a sexually transmitted infection and the need for notifying partners.
Patient: Feels embarrassed and worried, asks questions about treatment and next steps.

5. Communicating with Patients with Low Health Literacy:

Doctor: Explains a newly diagnosed chronic condition like diabetes, discusses management strategies.
Patient: Struggles to understand the implications of the diagnosis and how to manage the condition.

6. Importance of Adherence to Medication:

Pharmacist: Discusses the importance of adherence to antiretroviral therapy with a patient newly diagnosed with HIV.
Patient: Expresses concerns about side effects, managing medication

schedule, and impact on their lifestyle.

CHAPTER 2: RESPIRATORY CONDITIONS

I. Introduction
The respiratory system includes the nose, throat (pharynx), voice box (larynx), windpipe (trachea), bronchi, and lungs. It's responsible for taking in oxygen and expelling carbon dioxide. The process of gas exchange happens in the alveoli, small air sacs in the lungs.

II. Review of the Respiratory System
Upper Respiratory Tract: Includes the nasal cavity, pharynx, and larynx. This is often the first line of defense and the most common site for respiratory infections like the common cold.
Lower Respiratory Tract: Includes the trachea, bronchi, bronchioles, and alveoli. More serious infections like pneumonia can occur here.

Part 1: Cough

I. Introduction
Coughing is a vital defense mechanism that helps clear the airways of secretions, irritants, and foreign substances. It involves a quick intake of breath, closure of the vocal cords, and forceful release of air. Coughing can be triggered by many factors, including infections, allergies, asthma, and certain medications.

II. Understanding Types of Cough
A. Acute, Subacute, and Chronic Cough

1. **Acute Cough:** Lasts less than 3 weeks. Often caused by viral respiratory tract infections, such as the common cold or flu.
2. **Subacute Cough:** Lasts between 3 and 8 weeks. Common causes include post-infectious cough (following a cold or flu), bacterial sinusitis, or asthma.
3. **Chronic Cough:** Lasts more than 8 weeks. Common causes include chronic conditions such as asthma, gastroesophageal reflux disease (GERD), postnasal drip, chronic bronchitis, or lung diseases. In some cases, chronic cough could be a symptom of serious conditions like lung cancer or heart failure.

B. Causes of Different Types of Cough
Causes of Acute Cough:

1. Viral infections like the common cold or influenza.
2. Exposure to irritants such as smoke or dust.
3. Aspiration of food or liquids into the airways.
4. Acute bronchitis, often following a viral infection.

Causes of Subacute Cough:

1. Post-infectious cough, following a viral respiratory tract infection.
2. Bacterial sinusitis, an infection of the sinuses.
3. Asthma, especially if poorly controlled.

Causes of Chronic Cough:

1. Chronic conditions such as asthma, gastroesophageal reflux disease (GERD), and postnasal drip syndrome.
2. Chronic bronchitis, usually associated with smoking.
3. Lung diseases like pulmonary fibrosis or lung cancer.
4. Certain medications, particularly ACE inhibitors used for blood pressure control.
5. Heart failure, where a weak heart causes fluid build-up in the lungs.

III. Over-the-Counter (OTC) Treatments
A. Antitussives
Antitussives are medications used to suppress or relieve coughing. They work by blocking the cough reflex.
Common OTC Antitussives:

1. **Dextromethorphan**: A common OTC antitussive. It acts on the brain to suppress the cough reflex.
2. **Diphenhydramine:** An antihistamine with cough-suppressing effects.
3. **Codeine:** An opiate antitussives available OTC in some countries, but it has potential for misuse and dependence.

Usage and Side Effects:
Antitussives should be used as directed by the pharmacist or healthcare provider. Common side effects can include drowsiness, dizziness, nausea, and constipation. They should not be used in patients with chronic cough (e.g., due to asthma, COPD, or smoking), or in patients with a productive cough (as the suppression of cough can lead to mucus accumulation in the lungs).

Pharmacist Role:
Pharmacists can advise on the appropriate use of antitussives, including correct dosing and potential side effects. They can also guide the patient on when to seek further medical help if the cough persists or worsens, or if it is accompanied by other serious symptoms like high fever, chest pain, or shortness of breath.

B. Expectorants
Expectorants are medications that thin mucus in the airways, making it easier to cough up and clear. They can be helpful in treating coughs associated with conditions producing excessive mucus, such as

bronchitis.
Common OTC Expectorant:
Guaifenesin: A common OTC expectorant. It works by increasing the water content of mucus, thinning it and making it easier to cough up.
Usage and Side Effects:
Expectorants should be used as directed by the pharmacist or healthcare provider.
Common side effects can include nausea, vomiting, and stomach discomfort. These can be minimized by taking the medication with food. Adequate fluid intake is important when taking expectorants to help thin and loosen mucus.

C. Combination Products

Combination products contain more than one active ingredient. For coughs, these often include a combination of an antitussive, an expectorant, and/or a decongestant. Some may also contain pain relievers or antihistamines.
Common OTC Combination Products:
Examples include products containing dextromethorphan and guaifenesin, which act as a cough suppressant and an expectorant, respectively. Some products may also contain a decongestant like pseudoephedrine or phenylephrine.
Usage and Side Effects:
Combination products should be used as directed by the pharmacist or healthcare provider. Side effects depend on the specific components, but may include drowsiness, dizziness, nausea, vomiting, or increased heart rate. It's important to ensure that the medication is appropriate for the specific symptoms and that patients don't take multiple medications with overlapping ingredients.

Review of Common OTC Products and Their Active Ingredients

1. **Dextromethorphan (DM):** Found in products like Robitussin DM and Delsym. It's an antitussive, used to suppress a dry, nonproductive cough.
2. **Guaifenesin:** Found in products like Mucinex and Robitussin Chest Congestion. It's an expectorant, used to thin and loosen mucus in the airways, making it easier to cough up mucus and clear the airways.

3. **Diphenhydramine:** Found in products like Benadryl and ZzzQuil. It's an antihistamine with sedative effects, often used for allergies, but can also be used to relieve a cough.
4. **Pseudoephedrine and Phenylephrine:** Found in products like Sudafed (pseudoephedrine) and Sudafed PE (phenylephrine). They are decongestants, used to relieve nasal congestion associated with the common cold, sinusitis, or allergies.
5. **Combination Products:** Examples include Robitussin DM (dextromethorphan and guaifenesin), NyQuil (acetaminophen, dextromethorphan, and doxylamine), and Advil Cold & Sinus (ibuprofen and pseudoephedrine). These combine multiple active ingredients to address a range of symptoms.

IV. Patient Assessment and Recommendations
A. Asking the Right Questions:
When Did It Start?
This helps classify the cough as acute, subacute, or chronic, which can guide the treatment approach.
Dry or Productive?
A dry cough may benefit from antitussives to suppress the cough, while a productive cough may benefit from expectorants to help clear mucus.
Associated Symptoms?
Other symptoms can help identify the likely cause of the cough.
Fever or body aches may suggest an infection.
Wheezing or shortness of breath may suggest asthma or COPD.
Heartburn or a sour taste in the mouth may suggest GERD.
Other Important Questions:
Any known allergies or previous adverse reactions to medications?
Any other health conditions or current medications? Some conditions or medications may influence the choice of treatment.
Any lifestyle factors such as smoking or exposure to irritants?

B. Deciding on the Suitable Product Based on Symptoms and Patient's Medical History
Understanding Symptoms and Medical History:
Symptoms can suggest the type and cause of cough. For example, a dry, hacking cough might suggest a viral infection, while a productive cough could indicate bronchitis. The patient's medical history can impact treatment choices. For example, patients with high blood pressure should

avoid certain decongestants, and those with chronic cough due to asthma or COPD may require different treatments.

Product Selection:

1. **Dry cough**: An antitussive such as dextromethorphan.
2. **Productive cough**: An expectorant like guaifenesin.
3. **Cough with congestion**: A combination product with a decongestant.

Considerations:
It's essential to consider any potential interactions with the patient's current medications. The patient's age, pregnancy or breastfeeding status, and other health conditions should be taken into account.

C. Knowing When to Refer: Red Flags and Dangerous Symptoms

1. **High Fever or Severe Body Aches:** These may suggest a severe infection that requires medical attention.
2. **Cough Lasting More Than 3 Weeks:** This could indicate a chronic condition like asthma, GERD, or postnasal drip, or potentially serious conditions like lung cancer or heart failure.
3. **Shortness of Breath or Wheezing:** These could suggest asthma, COPD, or other serious lung conditions.
4. **Coughing up Blood or Pink, Frothy Sputum:** These are serious symptoms that require immediate medical attention.
5. **Unintentional Weight Loss, Night Sweats, or Fatigue:** These could be signs of serious conditions like tuberculosis or cancer.
6. **Chest Pain or Tightness:** This could suggest heart disease, especially if associated with exertion or stress.
7. **Exposure to Tuberculosis or Whooping Cough:** These infections require specific medical treatment.

Part 2: Common cold.

I. Introduction

The common cold is a viral infectious disease that primarily affects the upper respiratory tract, including the nose and throat. It is caused by a variety of viruses, with rhinoviruses being the most prevalent.
The common cold is recognized as the most frequent infectious disease in humans, with adults experiencing an average of 2-3 colds per year, and children suffering even more due to their developing immune systems. This widespread occurrence makes it a significant public health concern. While the common cold is generally mild and self-limiting, characterized by symptoms such as a runny nose, cough, and sore throat, it can have a notable impact on a patient's quality of life. Symptoms can lead to discomfort, disrupted daily activities, and absenteeism from work or school. Consequently, despite its benign nature, the common cold can result in substantial economic costs due to lost productivity and healthcare expenses.

Review of the Pathophysiology of the Common Cold
Viral Infection: The common cold is primarily caused by rhinoviruses, though other viruses like coronaviruses and influenza viruses can also be responsible. The virus typically enters through the nasal passages or through the eyes, attaching to the lining (mucosa) of the nose or throat.
Immune Response: Once a virus attaches to and invades cells, the body's immune system is activated. This response leads to inflammation and increased mucus production, which are responsible for the symptoms of the common cold.
Symptoms: Common symptoms include a runny or stuffy nose, sneezing, sore throat, mild headache, fatigue, and cough. Most people recover within 7-10 days, although some symptoms, like a cough, can last longer.
Spread: The common cold spreads through droplets in the air when someone with the cold coughs, sneezes, or talks. It can also spread by touching a surface or object that has the virus on it and then touching your own mouth, nose, or eyes.

II. Differentiating the Common Cold
A. Symptoms and Causes of the Common Cold

Symptoms of the Common Cold:

1. **Nasal Symptoms:** These are usually the first signs of a cold, and can include a runny nose, congestion, and sneezing.
2. **Throat Symptoms:** A sore or scratchy throat can occur as the cold progresses.
3. **Cough:** Coughing can develop later in the cold, often as a result of mucus dripping down the back of the throat.
4. **General Symptoms:** Other common symptoms can include mild headache, body aches, fatigue, and low-grade fever.

Causes of the Common Cold:
Viruses: The common cold is caused by several different viruses, with the most common being rhinoviruses. Other viruses that can cause colds include coronaviruses, parainfluenza viruses, and adenoviruses.
Transmission: The viruses that cause the common cold are spread through tiny air droplets that are released when a sick person sneezes, coughs, or blows their nose. You can get infected by inhaling these droplets or by touching a surface contaminated with them and then touching your face.
Distinguishing the Common Cold from Other Conditions:
Distinguishing Symptoms: Unlike the flu, the common cold usually comes on gradually and symptoms are generally mild. Allergies might cause similar symptoms to a cold, but they won't come with a fever or general malaise.
Duration of Illness: Colds usually last about 7-10 days. If symptoms persist beyond this, it may be an indication of a different condition, such as sinusitis or bronchitis, and the patient should seek medical attention.

B. Distinguishing Between the Common Cold, Flu, and Allergies

1. Common Cold:
Symptoms generally appear gradually over a few days. They often include a runny or stuffy nose, sneezing, mild headache, cough, sore throat, mild fatigue, and possibly a low-grade fever. They usually last about 7-10 days.

2. Influenza (Flu):
Symptoms often appear abruptly. They are more severe and can include high fever (usually 100.4°F/38°C or higher), severe fatigue, body aches, chills, dry cough, and sometimes gastrointestinal symptoms like nausea, vomiting, and diarrhea. Flu can lead to serious complications like pneumonia, especially in older adults, young children, pregnant women,

and people with chronic health conditions.

3. Allergies:

Symptoms can appear immediately after exposure to an allergen and can last as long as the person is exposed to it. They include runny or stuffy nose, sneezing, itchy or watery eyes, and sometimes a rash or hives. Unlike colds and flu, allergies do not cause fever. Seasonal allergies can occur in spring, summer, or fall, depending on what the individual is allergic to.

III. Over-the-Counter (OTC) Treatments

1. Decongestants

Decongestants are a type of medicine that can provide short-term relief for a blocked or stuffy nose (nasal congestion), which is often a symptom of a cold. They work by reducing swelling and inflammation in the nasal passages, thereby relieving congestion.

Types of Decongestants:

a. **Oral Decongestants:** Such as pseudoephedrine (Sudafed) and phenylephrine. These are used to relieve nasal and sinus congestion caused by colds and allergies. They are typically longer lasting but may have more systemic side effects.

b. **Topical Nasal Decongestants:** Such as oxymetazoline (Afrin) and phenylephrine (Neo-Synephrine). These provide quick relief directly to the nasal passages but should not be used for more than 3 days to avoid rebound congestion (rhinitis medicamentosa).

Side Effects:

Decongestants can cause restlessness, insomnia, or palpitations, particularly in people with cardiovascular disease, and should be used with caution in these patients. They can also raise blood pressure, so they should be avoided in people with uncontrolled high blood pressure.

Interactions:

Decongestants can interact with other medications including certain antidepressants, high blood pressure medications, and others. Always ask about other medications the patient is taking before recommending a decongestant.

2. Antihistamines

Antihistamines are often used to manage symptoms of allergies, but they can also provide some relief for symptoms of the common cold. They work by blocking the effects of histamine, a substance in the body that causes allergic symptoms.

Types of Antihistamines:

a. **First-Generation Antihistamines:** These include diphenhydramine (Benadryl) and chlorpheniramine. They are known for their sedating properties and can help with sleep in cases where the cold symptoms are preventing a good night's rest. They can also help with runny nose and sneezing.

b. **Second-Generation Antihistamines:** These include loratadine (Claritin), cetirizine (Zyrtec), and fexofenadine (Allegra). They are less sedating and are typically used for allergy symptoms but may provide some relief for cold symptoms.

Side Effects:
First-generation antihistamines can cause sedation, dry mouth, blurred vision, constipation, and urinary retention. Caution should be used in older adults due to the potential for falls and confusion. Second-generation antihistamines are less likely to cause sedation and other side effects, but they may not be as effective for cold symptoms.

Interactions:
Antihistamines can interact with several other types of medications, including certain antidepressants, some types of pain medication, and some antifungal and antiviral medications. Always confirm the other medications the patient is taking before recommending an antihistamine.

3. Pain Relievers

Pain relievers, also known as analgesics, can be used to manage symptoms such as sore throat, headache, and body aches that are often associated with the common cold.

Types of Pain Relievers:

a. **Acetaminophen (Tylenol):** Can relieve minor aches and pains, and reduce fever. It's generally safe for most people when used as directed, but high doses may cause liver damage.

b. **Nonsteroidal Anti-Inflammatory Drugs (NSAIDs):** These include ibuprofen (Advil, Motrin) and naproxen (Aleve). They can relieve pain and reduce inflammation and fever. They should be used with caution in people with stomach problems, kidney disease, heart disease, or high blood pressure, and those taking blood thinners.

Side Effects:
Acetaminophen is generally well-tolerated, but high doses can lead to liver toxicity.
NSAIDs can cause gastrointestinal upset, and with long-term use, can increase the risk of stomach ulcers and kidney or heart problems.

Interactions:
Both acetaminophen and NSAIDs can interact with other medications. For instance, they may increase the risk of bleeding when taken with blood thinners. NSAIDs can also decrease the effectiveness of certain blood pressure medications. Always ask about other medications the patient is taking before recommending a pain reliever.

4. Cough Suppressants

Cough suppressants, also known as antitussives, can help reduce or relieve the symptom of cough, which is common in the later stages of the common cold.

Types of Cough Suppressants:

a. **Dextromethorphan (DM):** This is a common OTC cough suppressant found in many multi-symptom cold remedies. It can help suppress the urge to cough.
b. **Codeine and Hydrocodone:** These are stronger cough suppressants that are available in some regions by prescription. They should be used for short periods of time under a healthcare provider's supervision due to their potential for side effects and dependence.

Side Effects:
Dextromethorphan can cause dizziness, gastrointestinal upset, and, in high doses, can lead to a feeling of disorientation or confusion. Codeine and hydrocodone can cause drowsiness, constipation, and have a risk of dependence with prolonged use.

Interactions:
Cough suppressants can interact with other medications, including some antidepressants, certain pain medications, and some drugs used for psychiatric conditions. Always ask about other medications the patient is taking before recommending a cough suppressant.

Review of Common OTC Products and Their Active Ingredients

When it comes to over-the-counter products for the common cold, it's important to understand that many products are combination products that contain more than one active ingredient. Here's a review of some common OTC products and their active ingredients:

1. **Tylenol Cold & Flu Severe:** Contains acetaminophen (pain reliever/fever reducer), dextromethorphan (cough suppressant), guaifenesin (expectorant), and phenylephrine (decongestant).
2. **Robitussin DM:** Contains dextromethorphan (cough suppressant) and guaifenesin (expectorant).
3. **Benadryl:** Contains diphenhydramine, a first-generation antihistamine.
4. **Zyrtec:** Contains cetirizine, a second-generation antihistamine.
5. **Claritin:** Contains loratadine, a second-generation antihistamine.
6. **Advil Cold & Sinus:** Contains ibuprofen (pain reliever/fever reducer) and pseudoephedrine (decongestant).
7. **Alka-Seltzer Plus Cold:** Contains aspirin (pain reliever/fever reducer), chlorpheniramine (antihistamine), and phenylephrine (decongestant).
8. **Mucinex DM:** Contains guaifenesin (expectorant) and dextromethorphan (cough suppressant).
9. **Sudafed PE:** Contains phenylephrine, a decongestant.
10. **Afrin Nasal Spray:** Contains oxymetazoline, a topical decongestant.

IV. Patient Assessment and Recommendations
A. Asking the Right Questions:

Before recommending any over-the-counter (OTC) treatments for cold, flu, or allergy symptoms, it's crucial to conduct a thorough patient assessment. Here are some key questions you need to ask:

Duration of Symptoms:
How long have you had these symptoms?
Have they been getting worse, better, or staying the same?
Colds and the flu usually resolve on their own within 1-2 weeks. If symptoms persist beyond this period, it could signal a more serious condition or complications. Allergy symptoms can last as long as the person is exposed to the allergen.

Symptoms:
What specific symptoms are you experiencing?
How severe are these symptoms?
The types of symptoms and their severity can help distinguish between a cold, the flu, and allergies. For example, high fever and body aches are more common with the flu, while itchy eyes and sneezing may suggest allergies.

Other Medications:
Are you currently taking any other medications, either prescription or over-the-counter?
This can help identify potential drug interactions. For example, decongestants can interact with certain antidepressants and blood pressure medications, and antihistamines can interact with certain pain medications.

Chronic Conditions:
Do you have any chronic health conditions, such as heart disease, high blood pressure, liver disease, kidney disease, or diabetes?
Certain OTC medications may not be suitable for people with specific chronic conditions. For example, decongestants can raise blood pressure, so they should be avoided in people with uncontrolled high blood pressure.

After gathering this information, you can then make an informed recommendation for treatment. Always advise patients to seek medical attention if their symptoms are severe, persist beyond a couple of weeks, or they have a high-risk condition that could lead to complications.

B. Recommending Suitable Products Based on Symptoms and Patient's Medical History

When recommending OTC products, it's crucial to match the active ingredients in the product to the patient's specific symptoms, while considering their overall health and other medications they are taking to avoid interactions and unnecessary side effects.

Here are some examples:

1. **For a patient with a runny nose and sneezing due to allergies, but no other symptoms:** An antihistamine like Claritin (loratadine), Zyrtec (cetirizine), or Allegra (fexofenadine) could be recommended. These second-generation antihistamines are less likely to cause drowsiness.
2. **For a patient with a blocked nose and sinus pressure from a cold, but with high blood pressure:** A decongestant like

pseudoephedrine (Sudafed) should be avoided due to its potential to increase blood pressure. A safer alternative might be a topical nasal decongestant like oxymetazoline (Afrin), but for no more than 3 days to avoid rebound congestion. You could also recommend a saline nasal spray for a safe and non-medicated option.

3. **For a patient with a sore throat and body aches from the flu:** Acetaminophen (Tylenol) could be recommended for its analgesic and antipyretic properties. If the patient has no contraindications, ibuprofen (Advil, Motrin) could also be an option.
4. **For a patient with a persistent, dry cough:** A cough suppressant like dextromethorphan (DM) could be recommended. If the cough is productive (bringing up mucus), an expectorant like guaifenesin might be more helpful.

C. Advice on Symptom Relief and When to See a Doctor

Beyond medication, there are several measures that can help alleviate symptoms and promote recovery:

1. **Rest and Hydration:** Rest allows the body to focus its energy on fighting off the virus, while staying well-hydrated helps thin mucus and soothe a sore throat.
2. **Warm Liquids:** Warm teas, soups, or broths can help soothe a sore throat and clear up congestion.
3. **Humidifier:** A humidifier can help keep the throat and nasal passages moist, which can alleviate congestion and coughing.
4. **Saline Nasal Spray or Rinse:** These can help clear the nasal passages of mucus and allergens.
5. **Avoid Allergens and Irritants:** If symptoms are due to allergies, it's important to avoid exposure to the triggering allergen when possible. This could include dust, pollen, pet dander, or certain foods.

In terms of when to see a doctor, advise patients to seek medical attention if:

1. Symptoms persist beyond two weeks or get worse instead of better.
2. They have high fever (>101.3 F or 38.5 C) for more than 3 days or a fever with a rash.

3. They experience severe symptoms such as difficulty breathing, chest pain, fainting, or confusion.
4. They have a chronic condition like asthma, heart disease, or diabetes, which could put them at risk of complications.

Chapter Summary

In this chapter, we discussed the common respiratory conditions that pharmacists frequently encounter, including coughs and the common cold.

Key points covered include:
1. Types of Cough: Distinguishing between acute, subacute, and chronic coughs to determine the appropriate treatment approach.
2. OTC Treatments for Cough: The use of antitussives (e.g., dextromethorphan) for dry coughs and expectorants (e.g., guaifenesin) for productive coughs.
3. Common Cold Management: Identifying the symptoms of the common cold and distinguishing it from flu and allergies, while recommending appropriate decongestants, antihistamines, and combination products.

Practical Activity
A. Case Studies

Case Study 1:
Patient: 30-year-old non-smoker with a week-long history of dry cough, runny nose, and low-grade fever.
Recommendation: Antitussive (e.g., dextromethorphan) for cough relief, and a decongestant for the runny nose. Advise the patient to rest, hydrate, and monitor symptoms.

Case Study 2:
Patient: 50-year-old smoker with a productive cough and shortness of breath lasting for a month.
Recommendation: This patient's cough could be due to a chronic condition like COPD, especially given the smoking history. The patient should be referred to a healthcare provider for further evaluation.

Case Study 3:
Patient: 25-year-old with a week-long history of productive cough and nasal congestion, no fever.
Recommendation: A combination product containing an expectorant (e.g., guaifenesin) and a decongestant. Advise the patient to rest, hydrate, and monitor symptoms.

Case Study 4:
Patient: 65-year-old with a history of high blood pressure, complaining of a cough with congestion.
Recommendation: A combination product containing an antitussive and an expectorant, but without a decongestant, as certain decongestants can raise blood pressure.

Case Study 5:
A 30-year-old woman comes in complaining of a runny nose, sneezing, and itchy eyes for the past two weeks. She states she has no known allergies and is not taking any medications.
Recommendation: Given the duration and symptoms, this may be seasonal allergies. An over-the-counter second-generation antihistamine like loratadine (Claritin), cetirizine (Zyrtec), or fexofenadine (Allegra) could be recommended. These are less likely to cause drowsiness.

Case Study 6:
A 50-year-old man with high blood pressure and a history of stomach ulcers presents with a headache and sinus congestion. He is currently taking a beta-blocker and a proton pump inhibitor.
Recommendation: Acetaminophen (Tylenol) can be used for the

headache as it doesn't carry the same risk of stomach irritation as NSAIDs. A topical nasal decongestant like oxymetazoline (Afrin) could be recommended for the congestion. However, it should not be used for more than 3 days to avoid rebound congestion. Oral decongestants are not recommended due to his high blood pressure.

Case Study 7:
A 25-year-old woman presents with a cough and body aches for the past three days. She also mentions having a fever. She is not on any medications and has no chronic conditions.

Recommendation: Given her symptoms of body aches, fever, and a cough, she may be experiencing the flu. Acetaminophen (Tylenol) can be recommended for pain and fever. A cough suppressant like dextromethorphan could be used for the cough. However, she should be advised to seek medical attention if her symptoms worsen or persist for more than a week.

B. Recommend OTC Products or Refer Based on Each Scenario

Scenario 1:
Patient: 45-year-old with a dry, hacking cough that's been going on for 3 days, no fever or other symptoms, known allergy to dextromethorphan.

Scenario 2:
Patient: 35-year-old with a productive cough that's been present for 10 days, also complaining of sinus pressure and a runny nose.

Scenario 3:
Patient: 55-year-old smoker with a cough that's been present for more than 3 weeks, also experiencing shortness of breath and a wheezing sound when breathing.

Scenario 4:
Patient: 70-year-old with a cough and congestion, also experiencing chest pain and tightness.

Scenario 5:
A 65-year-old man with diabetes and high blood pressure complains of a persistent cough and chest congestion. He is currently taking metformin for diabetes and lisinopril for hypertension.

Scenario 6:
A 25-year-old woman presents with symptoms of a runny nose, sneezing, itchy and watery eyes for a month. She is currently not taking any other medications.

Scenario 7:

A 35-year-old man is complaining of a severe sore throat, difficulty swallowing, and a high fever for the past two days. He also mentions a rash. He is currently not on any medications and has no known allergies.

CHAPTER 3: GASTROINTESTINAL HEALTH

I. Introduction
Overview of the Gastrointestinal Tract and the Mechanism of Digestion.

A. The Gastrointestinal Tract
Gastrointestinal Tract (GI Tract): The GI tract is a series of hollow organs joined in a long, twisting tube from the mouth to the anus. The main functions of the GI tract are digestion, absorption of nutrients, and excretion of waste products.

Parts of the GI Tract: The major parts include the mouth, esophagus, stomach, small intestine, and large intestine (which includes the rectum and anus).

Accessory Organs: The liver, gallbladder, and pancreas are accessory organs that contribute to digestion but are not part of the digestive tube.

B. The Mechanism of Digestion
The gastrointestinal tract, also known as the digestive tract, is a complex system that plays a critical role in the process of digestion and absorption of nutrients. Here's a brief overview:

1. **Mouth and Esophagus:** Digestion begins in the mouth where food is broken down into smaller pieces by chewing and mixed with saliva. The food then travels down the esophagus into the stomach through a process called peristalsis.
2. **Stomach:** The stomach secretes acid and enzymes that continue to break down the food into a semi-liquid substance called chyme.

3. **Small Intestine:** The chyme then moves into the small intestine, which is the major site for digestion and absorption of nutrients. Here, pancreatic enzymes and bile from the liver further break down the food particles. The walls of the small intestine are lined with villi and microvilli, tiny finger-like projections that increase the surface area for absorption.
4. **Large Intestine (Colon):** The large intestine absorbs water and electrolytes from the remaining indigestible food matter, and processes waste material (feces) for elimination.
5. **Rectum and Anus:** The waste material is then passed to the rectum and finally eliminated through the anus.

The entire process of digestion, from ingestion to excretion, is controlled by the nervous and hormonal systems, which coordinate the function of different organs and glands.

It's important to note that any disruption in this process, due to factors like disease, stress, or diet, can lead to gastrointestinal issues such as constipation, diarrhea, and irritable bowel syndrome (IBS).

Part 1: Constipation

I. Introduction
Overview of the Mechanism of Bowel Movements

1. **Digestion and Absorption:** Food is broken down in the stomach and small intestine, and nutrients are absorbed in the small intestine.
2. **Formation of Feces:** The remaining undigested material, water, and dead cells from the lining of the GI tract move into the large intestine, where they become stool.
3. **Defecation:** The rectum stores stool until it pushes it out of the body during a bowel movement.
4. **Muscle Contractions (Peristalsis):** Smooth muscles in the walls of the GI tract contract and relax in a coordinated rhythm to move food and waste through the system.

II. Understanding Constipation
A. Definition and Symptoms

Definition: Constipation is a common condition that affects the digestive system. It is characterized by infrequent bowel movements and difficulty in passing stools.

Symptoms: Here are some of the common symptoms associated with constipation:

1. Infrequent bowel movements: Fewer than three bowel movements per week.
2. Hard or lumpy stools: Difficulty or discomfort when passing stools.
3. Feeling of incomplete evacuation: The sensation of not being able to empty the stool from the bowels.
4. Straining to have bowel movements.
5. Abdominal bloating, cramps or pain.
6. Decreased appetite.

B. Common Causes and Risk Factors

Causes: It usually occurs when the colon absorbs too much water from the food that is in the colon, making the stools become hard and dry. This can be due to:

1. Slow transit: When the muscle contractions in the colon are slow or sluggish, causing the stool to move through the colon too slowly.
2. Pelvic floor dysfunction: Muscles of the pelvic floor fail to function properly and can interfere with the process of passing stool.

Risk Factors: Several factors can increase the likelihood of experiencing constipation:

1. **Inadequate fiber and fluid intake**: A diet low in fiber and not drinking enough fluids can contribute to constipation.
2. **Lack of physical activity**: Being sedentary can lead to constipation.
3. **Age**: Older adults are more likely to experience constipation, partly due to physical activity levels, dietary factors, and increased use of medications.
4. **Medications**: Certain medications, such as opioids, some antidepressants, certain antacids, and blood pressure medications, can cause constipation.
5. **Pregnancy**: Hormonal changes or pressure on the intestines from the growing uterus can lead to constipation in pregnant women.
6. **Ignoring the urge to have a bowel movement**: Habitually ignoring the need to go can contribute to constipation over time.

III. Over-the-Counter (OTC) Treatments
1. Bulk-Forming Laxatives

Definition: These are types of laxatives that work by increasing the water content and bulk of the stool, which helps to move it quickly through the colon. They are also known as fiber supplements and are often used for mild to moderate constipation.

Mechanism of Action: Bulk-forming laxatives absorb water in the intestine, swelling to form a soft, bulky stool. The increased bulk stimulates the intestinal reflexes and hastens bowel movement.

Examples: Some common bulk-forming laxatives include psyllium (Metamucil), methylcellulose (Citrucel), calcium polycarbophil (FiberCon), and wheat dextrin (Benefiber).

Usage: They are generally safe for long-term use and are often the first type of medication recommended for constipation relief. They should be

taken with plenty of water.
Side Effects: Side effects may include bloating, gas, cramping, or increased constipation if not taken with enough water.

2. Stimulant Laxatives

Definition: Stimulant laxatives are a type of laxative that works by increasing the contraction of muscles in the intestines, helping to promote bowel movements.
Mechanism of Action: These laxatives stimulate the nerves in the colon which increases its muscle contractions, and helps to move the stools along.
Examples: Common examples include bisacodyl (Dulcolax, Correctol), sennosides (Senokot, Ex-Lax), and castor oil.
Usage: While they are effective in relieving constipation, they are generally recommended for short-term use because they can lead to dependency if used regularly. They are often used when immediate or thorough bowel evacuation is needed.
Side Effects: Side effects may include abdominal cramping, diarrhea, nausea, vomiting, electrolyte imbalance and rectal irritation. Long-term use can also lead to decreased bowel function and dependency for bowel movements.

3. Osmotic Laxatives

Definition: Osmotic laxatives are a type of laxative that work by increasing the amount of water in the gut, softening the stool and making it easier to pass.
Mechanism of Action: These laxatives draw water into the intestines from the surrounding tissues, increasing the softness and volume of the stools. This increased volume stimulates the colon to contract and hasten bowel movement.
Examples: Common examples include polyethylene glycol (MiraLAX), lactulose (Kristalose), and magnesium salts (such as Milk of Magnesia).
Usage: Osmotic laxatives can be used for both immediate relief and longer-term management of constipation, though they typically take 1-3 days to work. They should be used with caution in elderly or debilitated patients or those with renal impairment.
Side Effects: Side effects may include bloating, gas, cramping, diarrhea, increased thirst, and electrolyte imbalances with prolonged use.
In recommending osmotic laxatives, pharmacists should remind patients to maintain proper hydration, as these medications can lead to increased

thirst and dehydration. It's also crucial to consider the patient's kidney function and other health conditions that may be affected by changes in electrolyte levels.

4. Stool Softeners

Definition: Stool softeners, also known as emollient laxatives, are a type of laxative that work by increasing the amount of water the stool absorbs in the gut, making the stool softer and easier to pass.

Mechanism of Action: These laxatives contain a compound called docusate, which increases the amount of water absorbed by the stools, making them softer and easier to pass.

Examples: Common examples include docusate sodium (Colace) and docusate calcium (Surfak).

Usage: Stool softeners are generally suggested for short-term use to alleviate constipation due to temporary circumstances, such as post-surgery or childbirth. They are often used when straining should be avoided (e.g., after a heart attack or surgery).

Side Effects: Side effects are usually mild but may include stomach cramps, diarrhea, or throat irritation (from the liquid form).

Stool softeners are generally considered safe for most patients, but they should be used as directed and not for extended periods. If constipation continues, patients should be advised to seek medical advice as prolonged constipation may be a symptom of a more serious condition. Pharmacists should also remind patients that stool softeners don't immediately relieve constipation — they usually work within 12 to 72 hours.

Review of Common OTC Products and Their Active Ingredients

1. **Bulk-Forming Laxatives:**

    Metamucil: Psyllium husk
    Citrucel: Methylcellulose
    FiberCon: Calcium polycarbophil
    Benefiber: Wheat dextrin

2. **Stimulant Laxatives:**

    Dulcolax, Correctol: Bisacodyl
    Senokot, Ex-Lax: Sennosides

Castor Oil

3. **Osmotic Laxatives:**

   MiraLAX: Polyethylene glycol 3350
   Kristalose: Lactulose
   Milk of Magnesia: Magnesium hydroxide

4. **Stool Softeners:**

   Colace, DulcoEase: Docusate Sodium
   Surfak: Docusate Calcium

Each of these products has its place in the management of constipation, depending on the patient's symptoms, the duration of their constipation, their overall health status, and other medications they may be taking. As a pharmacist, understanding the active ingredients and how they work can help you make the best recommendations for your patients.

IV. Patient Assessment and Recommendations
A. Asking the Right Questions:

When assessing a patient complaining of constipation, it's important to ask the right questions, as this can significantly aid in determining the most appropriate recommendation. Here are some key areas to explore:

1. **Duration of Symptoms:** How long has the patient been experiencing constipation? If the constipation is new or has been present for a prolonged period, it may warrant further medical evaluation.
2. **Severity of Symptoms:** How severe are the symptoms? Are they causing significant discomfort or distress? The severity can help determine the urgency and type of treatment required.
3. **Dietary Intake:** What does the patient's diet typically consist of? A diet low in fiber and fluids can often contribute to constipation.
4. **Physical Activity:** What is the patient's level of physical activity? Regular exercise can help stimulate normal bowel function.
5. **Medication History:** What medications, including over-the-counter drugs and supplements, is the patient currently taking? Certain medications can cause constipation.

For mild, short-term constipation, an over-the-counter laxative may be appropriate. In cases where the patient has dietary deficiencies or lacks physical activity, recommending dietary changes or more exercise may be beneficial.

For severe or chronic constipation, or if the patient is taking medications known to cause constipation, referral to a healthcare provider may be necessary.

B. Recommending Suitable Products Based on Symptoms and Patient's Medical History

In recommending a suitable product for constipation, it's important to consider both the patient's symptoms and medical history. Here are some general guidelines:

1. **Bulk-Forming Laxative:** If a patient's diet is low in fiber, a bulk-forming laxative like Metamucil or Benefiber might be a good first choice. These are also a good option for older adults or individuals who need to avoid straining. However, these are not suitable for patients with bowel obstruction or having difficulty swallowing.
2. **Stimulant Laxative:** For patients who need quick relief or have been unresponsive to other types of laxatives, a stimulant laxative like Dulcolax or Senokot might be appropriate. However, these should not be used long-term without a doctor's supervision and are not suitable for patients with bowel obstruction.
3. **Osmotic Laxative:** If a patient needs more than just fiber supplementation, an osmotic laxative like MiraLAX or Milk of Magnesia might be suitable. These are often used for short-term relief but can also be used for chronic constipation under medical supervision. They are not recommended for patients with kidney disease or heart failure.
4. **Stool Softener:** For patients who should avoid straining, such as those recovering from surgery or childbirth, a stool softener like Colace could be recommended.

Remember, if a patient has been using OTC laxatives regularly without relief, has blood in their stool, or has lost weight unexpectedly, these could be signs of a more serious underlying condition. In these cases, it's important to refer the patient to a healthcare provider for further evaluation. Lastly, it's a good practice to remind patients that lifestyle modifications such as eating a high-fiber diet, staying well-hydrated, and getting regular exercise are vital in managing constipation.

C. Providing Lifestyle and Dietary Advice

While medications can be effective for relieving symptoms of constipation, it's also crucial to provide patients with advice on lifestyle and dietary changes that can help prevent constipation in the long term. Here are some recommendations:

1. **Increase Fiber Intake:** A diet high in fiber can add bulk and volume to stools, making them easier to pass. Recommend consuming more fruits, vegetables, whole grains, and legumes.
2. **Stay Hydrated:** Drinking plenty of fluids can help prevent dehydration, which can cause constipation. Water is the best choice, but fruit juices (especially prune juice) can also be helpful.
3. **Regular Exercise:** Regular physical activity can stimulate the muscles in the intestines, helping to move stools through the digestive system.
4. **Don't Ignore the Urge:** Encourage patients not to ignore the urge to have a bowel movement. Over time, ignoring the urge can lead to constipation.
5. **Establish a Routine:** Having a regular routine for bowel movements can also help some people manage constipation. This might involve setting aside time each day for a bowel movement, such as after a meal.
6. **Limit Foods That Cause Constipation:** Some people may find that certain foods lead to constipation. Common culprits include dairy products, processed foods, and foods high in fat and sugar.
7. **Limit Alcohol and Caffeine:** Both can lead to dehydration and might contribute to constipation.
8. **Quit Smoking:** Nicotine in cigarettes can contribute to constipation, so quitting smoking can help relieve symptoms.

Remember to remind patients that results from these changes may not be immediate and consistency is key. If these lifestyle and dietary changes don't help or if symptoms worsen, they should seek additional medical advice.

D. Recognizing When to Refer: Red Flags and Serious Symptoms

While many cases of constipation can be managed with over-the-counter (OTC) medications and lifestyle changes, it's important to recognize when a patient needs to be referred to a healthcare provider for further evaluation. Here are some red flags and serious symptoms that warrant a referral:

1. **Duration of Symptoms:** If a patient has been constipated for an extended period (more than three weeks) without relief from OTC treatments, they should be referred to a healthcare provider.
2. **Blood in Stool:** This can be a sign of a more serious condition, such as colorectal cancer.
3. **Severe Abdominal Pain:** While some discomfort is common with constipation, severe or persistent abdominal pain could indicate a more serious issue, such as an intestinal blockage.
4. **Sudden Change in Bowel Habits:** If a patient over the age of 50 experiences a sudden change in bowel habits, this could be a sign of colorectal cancer and should be evaluated by a healthcare provider.
5. **Unexpected Weight Loss:** Losing weight without trying can be a sign of many serious health conditions, including cancer.
6. **Family History:** A family history of certain diseases, including colorectal cancer or inflammatory bowel disease, may necessitate a referral, especially if the patient is experiencing ongoing constipation.
7. **Presence of Other Symptoms:** If the patient is also experiencing symptoms such as vomiting, fever, or severe bloating, it's important to refer them to a healthcare provider.
8. **Failure to Respond to Treatment:** If a patient's symptoms do not improve after a week of treatment with OTC laxatives, they should be referred to a healthcare provider.
9. **Frequent Need for Laxatives:** If a person needs to use laxatives regularly to have a bowel movement, it suggests that they need medical evaluation to identify any underlying issues.

Part 2: Diarrhea

I. Introduction

Diarrhea is a common gastrointestinal condition characterized by the frequent passage of loose or watery stools. It can range from a mild, self-limiting condition to a severe and potentially life-threatening problem, particularly in vulnerable populations such as young children, the elderly, and immunocompromised individuals.

In community pharmacy practice, pharmacists often encounter patients seeking advice on managing diarrhea, whether it's due to infections, dietary indiscretions, medication side effects, or underlying health conditions. A thorough understanding of the causes, symptoms, and treatment options for diarrhea is essential for providing effective patient care.

This section will cover the key aspects of diarrhea, including common causes, over-the-counter treatments, and when to refer patients to healthcare providers for further evaluation. By equipping pharmacists with practical tools and advice, we aim to improve patient outcomes and ensure proper management of this common condition.

II. Understanding Diarrhea
A. Definition and Symptoms
Definition
Diarrhea is characterized by loose or watery stools that occur three or more times in a day. It's a common condition that often lasts a couple of days and usually isn't serious.

Symptoms of Diarrhea include:

1. Frequent loose, watery stools.
2. Abdominal cramps.
3. Bloating.
4. Urgent need to have a bowel movement.
5. Nausea.
6. Dehydration symptoms such as thirst, less frequent urination, dark-colored urine, fatigue, and light-headedness.

Symptoms can be mild or severe and can have a significant impact on quality of life. It's important to note that these symptoms can also be signs of other, more serious conditions, so it's essential to consult a healthcare professional if symptoms persist, worsen, or are accompanied by other worrying signs like blood in the stool or unexplained weight loss.

B. Common Causes and Risk Factors

Diarrhea can be caused by a number of factors, including:

1. **Infections:** Bacterial, viral, or parasitic infections can cause diarrhea. These infections can be caught from food poisoning, contaminated water, or from another person with the infection.
2. **Food intolerances and sensitivities:** Some people are sensitive to certain types of food such as dairy products (lactose intolerance) or artificial sweeteners, which can cause diarrhea.
3. **Medications:** Certain medicines, such as antibiotics, can trigger diarrhea by disturbing the natural balance of bacteria in your intestines.
4. **Gastrointestinal disorders:** Conditions like irritable bowel syndrome (IBS), inflammatory bowel disease (IBD), celiac disease, and Crohn's disease can lead to frequent bouts of diarrhea.

III. Over-the-Counter (OTC) Treatments
Antidiarrheal Medications

OTC treatments can be very effective for the management of acute diarrhea and the relief of IBS symptoms. Here are some commonly used antidiarrheal medications:

1. **Loperamide (Imodium):** This slows down the movement of the gut. This allows more time for water and electrolytes to be absorbed back into the body, resulting in firmer stools that are passed less often.
2. **Bismuth subsalicylate (Pepto-Bismol):** This medication can reduce the frequency of stools and relieve abdominal cramping. It also has antimicrobial properties which can be beneficial if the diarrhea is caused by an infection.
3. **Probiotics:** Certain types of probiotics have been found to help regulate the digestive system and can reduce the duration of diarrhea, particularly when it is caused by antibiotics.

Remember, OTC medicines should only be used as directed, and it is important to read the label carefully to check for any contraindications or potential side effects. For persistent or severe symptoms, medical advice should be sought.

It's also worth mentioning that OTC treatments are not a substitute for rehydration. Oral rehydration solutions, which are also available over the counter, should be used in conjunction with antidiarrheal medications to prevent dehydration.

Dietary Supplements (Probiotics)

Probiotics are live bacteria and yeasts that are good for your health, especially your digestive system. Our bodies are full of bacteria, both good and bad. Probiotics are often called "good" or "friendly" bacteria because they help keep your gut healthy.

When it comes to managing gastrointestinal issues like diarrhea and IBS, certain strains of probiotics have been found to be beneficial:

1. **Lactobacillus and Bifidobacterium:** These are the most commonly used probiotics and have been shown to help with diarrhea and symptoms of IBS. They work by restoring the natural balance of bacteria in the gut.
2. **Saccharomyces boulardii:** This is a yeast found in probiotics that appears to help with diarrhea and other digestive problems.
3. **Bacillus coagulans:** This strain has been shown to help with abdominal pain and bloating in people with IBS.

Probiotics are generally considered safe for most people, but they can cause gas and bloating in some people. They are available in a variety of forms, including capsules, tablets, powders, and foods like yogurt. It's important to note that the potency and effectiveness of probiotics can vary significantly between products, and not all probiotics have the same effects. Therefore, it's important to choose a product that has been scientifically tested for the specific condition you're looking to treat.

Review of Common OTC Products and Their Active Ingredients

1. **Loperamide (Imodium):** This medication can help reduce the frequency of diarrhea. The active ingredient, loperamide, works by slowing down the movement of the gut.
2. **Bismuth subsalicylate (Pepto-Bismol):** This can be used to treat diarrhea and upset stomach. The active ingredient, bismuth

subsalicylate, can reduce inflammation, kill bacteria, and coat the stomach lining.

IV. Patient Assessment and Recommendations
A. Asking the Right Questions:
When a patient presents with symptoms of diarrhea, a thorough assessment is essential to provide appropriate recommendations. Here are key questions to ask:

1. **Duration of Symptoms:** How long has the patient been experiencing symptoms? Acute symptoms may indicate an infection or reaction to food or medication, while chronic symptoms may suggest a condition like IBS or other gastrointestinal disorders.
2. **Severity of Symptoms:** How many bowel movements does the patient have per day? Are they able to maintain their daily activities? Severe or debilitating symptoms may indicate a more serious condition that requires immediate medical attention.
3. **Associated Symptoms:** Are there any other symptoms present, such as blood in the stool, fever, weight loss, or severe abdominal pain? These may suggest a more serious condition.
4. **Dietary History:** Has the patient been eating any new foods or taking any new medications? This could help identify potential triggers for the symptoms.
5. **Stress Levels:** Has the patient been under significant stress recently? Stress can exacerbate symptoms.

Based on the assessment, you can provide recommendations:
If symptoms are severe, associated with other worrying symptoms, or persistent for a prolonged period, the patient should be referred for immediate medical attention. For acute diarrhea, over-the-counter medications like loperamide (Imodium) or bismuth subsalicylate (Pepto-Bismol) may be recommended, along with oral rehydration solutions to prevent dehydration.

B. Recommending Suitable OTC Products Based on Symptoms and Patient's Medical History
Recommending the right over-the-counter (OTC) products to a patient should be based on the symptoms they present, their medical history, and any other medications they are currently taking.

For Acute Diarrhea: If the patient does not have any warning signs such as fever, bloody stools, severe pain, or signs of dehydration, an OTC antidiarrheal like loperamide (Imodium) or bismuth subsalicylate (Pepto-Bismol) can be recommended. The patient should also be reminded of the importance of staying hydrated.

It's important to consider the patient's other health conditions and medications. For example, some antidiarrheals can interact with certain medications, and certain health conditions may contraindicate the use of some OTC products. Always recommend patients to consult with a healthcare professional before starting any new medication.

C. Providing Dietary and Lifestyle Advice

1. **Balanced Diet:** Encourage a balanced diet rich in fruits, vegetables, lean proteins, and whole grains. These foods provide necessary nutrients and fiber, which can help regulate bowel movements.
2. **Hydration:** Hydration is especially crucial in cases of diarrhea to prevent dehydration. Recommend drinking plenty of water and consider an oral rehydration solution for severe cases.
3. **Identify Triggers:** Advise keeping a food diary to identify potential trigger foods. Common triggers include dairy products, certain fruits and vegetables, grains, artificial sweeteners, alcohol, caffeine, and spicy foods.

D. Recognizing When to Refer: Red Flags and Serious Symptoms

It's important to recognize when symptoms may indicate a more serious condition and therefore require immediate medical attention. Here are some "red flags" and serious symptoms that warrant a referral to a healthcare professional:

1. **Duration of Symptoms:** If symptoms persist for more than a few weeks with no improvement despite self-management strategies, it's important to seek medical attention.
2. **Severe Pain:** Severe, persistent, or worsening abdominal pain should be evaluated by a healthcare professional.
3. **Weight Loss:** Unexplained weight loss could indicate a serious underlying condition such as inflammatory bowel disease (IBD) or even cancer.

4. **Blood in the Stool:** This could be a sign of bleeding in the digestive tract, which is a medical emergency.
5. **Fever:** Fever along with diarrhea could indicate a serious infection that needs urgent medical attention.
6. **Signs of Dehydration:** This includes excessive thirst, dry mouth, little or no urine or dark urine, severe weakness, dizziness, or lightheadedness.
7. **Age:** Elderly people and very young children are more at risk of complications from diarrhea, and should be evaluated by a healthcare professional.
8. **Other Health Conditions:** Those with weakened immune systems, such as people living with HIV/AIDS, those on chemotherapy, or those who have had organ transplants, should seek medical attention.
9. **Pregnancy:** If a pregnant woman experiences severe diarrhea, she should consult a healthcare provider.
10. **Travel History:** If the patient has recently traveled to a foreign country, particularly where sanitation is poor, and has developed diarrhea, they should seek medical attention to rule out conditions such as traveler's diarrhea or parasitic infections.

Part 3: Inflammatory Bowel Syndrome (IBS)

I. Introduction

Irritable Bowel Syndrome (IBS) is a common gastrointestinal disorder characterized by a group of symptoms that affect the large intestine. It is classified as a functional bowel disorder, meaning it involves a dysfunction of the bowel without any identifiable structural abnormalities.

IBS affects a significant portion of the population, with estimates suggesting that up to 15% of adults may experience symptoms at some point in their lives. The condition is more prevalent in women and often manifests in late adolescence or early adulthood.

While IBS is not life-threatening, it can substantially impact patients' quality of life. Many individuals struggle with the unpredictability of their symptoms, leading to anxiety, social withdrawal, and reduced productivity.

II. Understanding IBS
A. Definition and Symptoms
Definition

IBS is a common disorder that affects the large intestine. Unlike other inflammatory bowel diseases, IBS doesn't cause changes in bowel tissue or increase the risk of colorectal cancer.

Symptoms can vary widely but often include:

1. Abdominal pain or cramping that is often relieved by passing a bowel movement.
2. Changes in bowel habits — such as diarrhea, constipation, or alternating episodes of both.
3. Changes in the appearance of bowel movements.
4. Bloating or excess gas.
5. The feeling that you haven't completely emptied your bowels after a bowel movement.

Symptoms can be mild or severe and can have a significant impact on quality of life. It's important to note that these symptoms can also be signs of other, more serious conditions, so it's essential to consult a healthcare professional if symptoms persist, worsen, or are accompanied by other worrying signs like blood in the stool or unexplained weight loss.

B. Common Causes and Risk Factors

The exact cause of IBS isn't known, but several factors appear to play a role, including:

1. **Muscle contractions in the intestine:** The walls of the intestines are lined with layers of muscle that contract and relax as they move food from your stomach through your intestinal tract to your rectum. If these contractions are stronger and last longer than normal, you might have diarrhea.
2. **Nervous system abnormalities:** An overactive or underactive gut nervous system can cause pain, slow down or speed up gut motility, causing constipation or diarrhea.
3. **Severe infection:** IBS can develop after a severe bout of diarrhea (post-infectious IBS).
4. **Changes in gut microbiota:** This is the 'good' bacteria in the gut; changes in gut bacteria can influence IBS.

Risk Factors:
Factors that can increase a person's risk of developing IBS include:

1. **Young age:** IBS typically begins before the age of 50.
2. **Being female:** In some studies, women are twice as likely as men to have IBS.
3. **Family history:** Genes may play a role, as may shared factors in a family's environment or a combination of genes and environment.
4. **Mental health problems:** Anxiety, depression, a personality disorder, and a history of childhood sexual abuse are risk factors. For women, domestic abuse may be a risk factor as well.

III. Over-the-Counter (OTC) Treatments

The medications used to treat IBS depend on whether the main symptom is constipation, diarrhea, or both. Here are some of the common classes of medications used:

1. **Fiber Supplements:** Fiber can help control constipation by softening stool, making it easier to pass. An example is psyllium (Metamucil).
2. **Laxatives:** In some cases, over-the-counter laxatives may be recommended for short-term relief of constipation. These

include osmotic laxatives like polyethylene glycol (Miralax) and stimulant laxatives like senna (Sennakot).
3. **Antidiarrheals:** As mentioned before, loperamide (Imodium) can be used to help manage episodes of diarrhea in IBS.
4. **Antispasmodics:** These help to relieve abdominal cramping and pain by relaxing the muscles in the gut. Examples include dicyclomine (Bentyl) and hyoscyamine (Levsin).
5. **Medications that affect certain activities of the gut:** These include alosetron (Lotronex), which slows stool transit in the gut and is used in severe cases of IBS-D, and lubiprostone (Amitiza), which speeds up stool transit and is used in IBS-C.
6. **Antidepressants:** Low doses of certain types of antidepressants, such as tricyclic antidepressants and selective serotonin reuptake inhibitors (SSRIs), have been found to help with IBS symptoms.
7. **Probiotics:** As discussed earlier, certain types of probiotics may help with IBS symptoms.

While some of these medications are available over-the-counter, others require a prescription. Therefore, it's always important for patients to discuss their symptoms with a healthcare provider to determine the best treatment plan. Also, it's key to understand that while these medications can help manage symptoms, they do not cure IBS. A comprehensive approach that includes dietary and lifestyle changes is often most effective.

Review of Common OTC Products and Their Active Ingredients

1. **Psyllium (Metamucil):** This is a fiber supplement that can help regulate bowel movements, especially for those with IBS-C. The active ingredient, psyllium husk, absorbs water to form a gel-like substance, making the stool softer and larger.
2. **Polyethylene glycol 3350 (Miralax):** This is an osmotic laxative that helps to increase the amount of water in the intestinal tract to stimulate bowel movements.
3. **Dicyclomine (Bentyl):** This is an antispasmodic medication that helps to reduce intestinal spasms.
4. **Simethicone (Gas-X, Mylicon):** This medication is used to relieve symptoms of excess gas such as belching, bloating, and feelings of pressure/discomfort in the stomach/gut. Simethicone works by breaking up gas bubbles in the gut.

5. **Probiotic supplements:** These can come in many forms and contain a variety of different species and strains of beneficial bacteria, including Lactobacillus, Bifidobacterium, and Saccharomyces boulardii.

IV. Patient Assessment and Recommendations
A. Asking the Right Questions:

When a patient presents with symptoms of IBS, a thorough assessment is essential to provide appropriate recommendations. Here are key questions to ask:

1. **Duration of Symptoms:** How long has the patient been experiencing symptoms? Acute symptoms may indicate an infection or reaction to food or medication, while chronic symptoms may suggest a condition like IBS or other gastrointestinal disorders.
2. **Severity of Symptoms:** How many bowel movements does the patient have per day? Are they able to maintain their daily activities? Severe or debilitating symptoms may indicate a more serious condition that requires immediate medical attention.
3. **Associated Symptoms:** Are there any other symptoms present, such as blood in the stool, fever, weight loss, or severe abdominal pain? These may suggest a more serious condition.
4. **Dietary History:** Has the patient been eating any new foods or taking any new medications? This could help identify potential triggers for the symptoms.
5. **Stress Levels:** Has the patient been under significant stress recently? Stress can exacerbate symptoms of IBS and other digestive issues.

Based on the assessment, you can provide recommendations:

If symptoms are severe, associated with other worrying symptoms, or persistent for a prolonged period, the patient should be referred for immediate medical attention.

For those with symptoms suggestive of IBS, a comprehensive management approach that includes dietary modifications (such as a low FODMAP diet), stress management, and potentially medication may be needed. A referral to a healthcare professional is recommended to establish a diagnosis and management plan.

Probiotic supplements may be recommended for some patients,

depending on the nature of their symptoms and their dietary history.

B. Recommending Suitable OTC Products Based on Symptoms and Patient's Medical History

Recommending the right over-the-counter (OTC) products to a patient should be based on the symptoms they present, their medical history, and any other medications they are currently taking. Here are some common scenarios:

1. **IBS with Diarrhea (IBS-D):** For patients with diagnosed IBS-D, an antidiarrheal like loperamide can help manage symptoms. Probiotic supplements may also be considered, particularly those containing strains like Lactobacillus or Bifidobacterium which have been shown to improve IBS symptoms.
2. **IBS with Constipation (IBS-C):** A fiber supplement like psyllium (Metamucil) can help regulate bowel movements. An osmotic laxative such as polyethylene glycol (Miralax) may also be recommended for short-term relief of constipation.
3. **Gas and Bloating:** Products containing simethicone (Gas-X, Mylicon) can help relieve symptoms of excess gas.
4. **Stress-related IBS:** If the patient's symptoms seem to be exacerbated by stress, lifestyle modifications including regular exercise, adequate sleep, and stress management techniques should be recommended.

C. Providing Dietary and Lifestyle Advice

1. **Balanced Diet:** Encourage a balanced diet rich in fruits, vegetables, lean proteins, and whole grains. These foods provide necessary nutrients and fiber, which can help regulate bowel movements.
2. **Fiber Intake:** For those with constipation-predominant IBS, increasing dietary fiber intake can help. However, for some, too much fiber, especially insoluble fiber, can exacerbate bloating and gas.
3. **Low FODMAP Diet:** Some people with IBS find relief from a low FODMAP diet, which limits certain types of carbohydrates that can cause gas and bloating.
4. **Identify Triggers:** Advise keeping a food diary to identify potential trigger foods. Common triggers include dairy products,

certain fruits and vegetables, grains, artificial sweeteners, alcohol, caffeine, and spicy foods.

D. Lifestyle Advice:

1. **Regular Exercise:** Regular physical activity can help stimulate the muscles of the intestine and reduce constipation. It can also help reduce stress, a common trigger for IBS symptoms.
2. **Stress Management:** Techniques such as meditation, deep breathing exercises, yoga, and other relaxation practices can help manage stress levels, which can impact gut health.
3. **Adequate Sleep:** Encourage maintaining a regular sleep schedule. Disruptions in the sleep-wake cycle can exacerbate IBS symptoms.
4. **Limit Alcohol and Caffeine:** These can stimulate the intestines and can worsen diarrhea and other IBS symptoms.
5. **Quit Smoking:** Smoking can worsen digestive problems and increase the risk of various gastrointestinal diseases.
6. **Regular Health Checks:** Regular visits to a healthcare professional for check-ups can help monitor the condition and make necessary changes to the management plan.

It's important to note that everyone is different, and what works for one person might not work for another. Changes should be introduced slowly and one at a time, to monitor the effect they have on symptoms. As always, consult a healthcare professional before making significant changes to diet or lifestyle.

E. Recognizing When to Refer: Red Flags and Serious Symptoms

While many cases of diarrhea and IBS can be managed with over-the-counter treatments and lifestyle modifications, it's important to recognize when symptoms may indicate a more serious condition and therefore require immediate medical attention.

Here are some **"red flags"** and serious symptoms that warrant a referral to a healthcare professional:

1. **Duration of Symptoms:** If symptoms persist for more than a few weeks with no improvement despite self-management strategies, it's important to seek medical attention.

2. **Severe Pain:** Severe, persistent, or worsening abdominal pain should be evaluated by a healthcare professional.
3. **Weight Loss:** Unexplained weight loss could indicate a serious underlying condition such as inflammatory bowel disease (IBD) or even cancer.
4. **Blood in the Stool:** This could be a sign of bleeding in the digestive tract, which is a medical emergency.
5. **Fever:** Fever along with diarrhea could indicate a serious infection that needs urgent medical attention.
6. **Other Health Conditions:** Those with weakened immune systems, such as people living with HIV/AIDS, those on chemotherapy, or those who have had organ transplants, should seek medical attention.

Part 4: Gastroesophageal Reflux Disease GERD

I. Introduction
Overview of the Gastrointestinal Tract and the Mechanism of Reflux

The gastrointestinal (GI) tract, also known as the digestive tract, is a complex system that plays a crucial role in the body's ability to digest food, absorb nutrients, and expel waste. From ingestion to excretion, it includes the following major components:

1. **Mouth:** The entry point where food is ingested and the process of digestion begins with mechanical and chemical breakdown of food.
2. **Esophagus:** A muscular tube that connects the throat to the stomach and uses peristalsis (wave-like muscle contractions) to propel food downward.
3. **Stomach:** A sac-like organ that uses gastric acid and enzymes to further break down the food into a semi-fluid mass called chyme.
4. **Small Intestine:** The longest part of the GI tract where most digestion and absorption of nutrients occur. It is divided into three sections: the duodenum, jejunum, and ileum.
5. **Large Intestine (Colon):** Absorbs water and electrolytes from the remaining indigestible food matter and transmits the useless waste material from the body.
6. **Rectum and Anus:** The rectum stores feces until they can be eliminated through the anus.

Mechanism of Reflux:
Reflux, specifically Gastroesophageal Reflux Disease (GERD), occurs when stomach acid or, occasionally, stomach content, flows back into your food pipe (esophagus). The backwash (reflux) irritates the lining of your esophagus and causes GERD.

Both acid reflux and GERD are chronic conditions that occur when the muscle at the end of your esophagus (the lower esophageal sphincter or LES) doesn't close properly, allowing acid to rise up into the esophagus. This malfunction can be caused by a variety of factors such as obesity, smoking, certain medications, and foods like caffeine, alcohol, chocolate, and fatty or fried foods.

II. Understanding GERD

A. Definition and Symptoms

Definition:
Gastroesophageal Reflux Disease (GERD) is a chronic digestive disorder that occurs when stomach acid or, occasionally, bile, flows back (refluxes) into your food pipe (esophagus). This backwash (acid reflux) can irritate the lining of your esophagus, causing uncomfortable symptoms and potentially leading to more serious health complications.

Symptoms:
Symptoms of GERD can vary in severity and frequency from person to person. Some may experience mild symptoms occasionally, while others might experience severe, persistent symptoms. The most common symptoms include:

1. **Heartburn:** Also known as acid indigestion, heartburn is a burning pain or discomfort that can move up from your stomach to the middle of your abdomen and chest, and even up into your throat.
2. **Regurgitation:** This is another common symptom where a sour or bitter-tasting acid backs up into your throat or mouth.
3. **Dyspepsia:** People with GERD often experience dyspepsia, which is stomach discomfort, bloating, nausea after eating, stomach fullness or bloating, and upper abdominal pain and discomfort.
4. **Sore Throat or Hoarseness:** Chronic throat irritation, persistent cough or hoarseness, and difficulty swallowing can also be symptoms of GERD.
5. **Chest Pain:** If the esophagus goes into spasm, it can cause severe chest pain that can be mistaken for a heart attack.
6. **Sleep Problems:** GERD can cause problems with Eustachian tube function (connecting the pharynx to the middle ear) and problems with sleep.

It's important to note that some people with GERD may have atypical symptoms, such as coughing, asthma-like symptoms, or trouble swallowing, without experiencing heartburn. Also, individuals with long-standing GERD can develop complications such as esophageal stricture, Barrett's esophagus, and esophageal cancer.

B. Common Causes and Risk Factors

GERD is primarily caused by the dysfunction of the lower esophageal sphincter (LES), which normally acts as a barrier preventing the backflow of stomach contents into the esophagus. However, a combination of factors can contribute to the development of GERD. These include:

1. **Lower Esophageal Sphincter (LES) Abnormalities:** The LES is a ring of muscle at the bottom of the esophagus that acts like a valve between the esophagus and stomach. If this valve relaxes abnormally or weakens, acid can flow back into the esophagus, causing GERD.
2. **Hiatal Hernia:** A condition where the upper part of the stomach bulges through the large muscle separating the abdomen and chest (diaphragm). This structural abnormality can contribute to the development of GERD.
3. **Pregnancy:** Pregnancy can increase the risk of GERD, as hormonal changes and the physical pressure of a growing fetus can lead to acid reflux.
4. **Obesity:** Excess belly fat can put pressure on the stomach, causing the LES to relax and allow acid to reflux into the esophagus.
5. **Lifestyle Factors:** Certain lifestyle choices can increase the risk of GERD. These include smoking, alcohol consumption, eating large meals or eating late at night, eating certain types of food (such as fatty or fried foods, chocolate, caffeine, onions, mint), and certain medications (including aspirin, ibuprofen, certain muscle relaxers, or blood pressure medications).
6. **Other Medical Conditions:** Conditions like asthma, diabetes, and peptic ulcers can increase the risk of developing GERD.

It's essential to understand these causes and risk factors, as this knowledge is key to both prevention and management of GERD. In the next section, we'll delve into the potential complications if GERD is left untreated.

C. Complications if Left Untreated

If GERD is not managed properly, it can lead to a range of complications over time. These include:

1. **Esophagitis:** This is inflammation that can damage tissues of the esophagus, the muscular tube that delivers food from your mouth to your stomach. Continuous backwash of acid can irritate and inflame the lining of the esophagus.

2. **Esophageal Stricture:** Over time, the damage caused by stomach acid can lead to scar tissue that narrows the space inside the esophagus. This can make swallowing difficult.
3. **Barrett's Esophagus:** In this condition, the tissue lining the lower esophagus changes. These changes are associated with an increased risk of esophageal cancer.
4. **Esophageal Cancer:** Long-standing GERD can lead to certain types of esophageal cancer, especially in adults over 40 years old.
5. **Respiratory Problems:** GERD can cause respiratory problems such as pneumonia, bronchitis, and asthma. Acid from the stomach can be aspirated into the lungs, causing a variety of respiratory issues.
6. **Dental Problems:** GERD can also lead to dental problems. The acid can erode tooth enamel and increase the risk of cavities.

III. Over-the-Counter (OTC) Treatments
1. Antacids

Antacids are the most commonly used over-the-counter (OTC) treatment for mild intermittent heartburn and indigestion. They work by neutralizing the acid in your stomach to relieve symptoms of heartburn. Key points to cover in this section:

Mechanism of Action: Antacids work by chemically neutralizing gastric acid, which directly reduces the acidity in the stomach. They can provide quick, short-term relief for heartburn and indigestion symptoms.

Common Types: Common ingredients in antacids include magnesium (as in Milk of Magnesia), calcium carbonate (as in Tums), aluminum hydroxide (as in Maalox), and sodium bicarbonate (as in Alka-Seltzer).

Usage: Antacids are used to relieve heartburn, acid indigestion, sour stomach, and GERD symptoms. They are usually taken on an as-needed basis.

Side Effects: While generally safe, antacids can cause side effects such as diarrhea and constipation. Some antacids can also lead to an electrolyte imbalance (particularly in magnesium and calcium levels) if taken in large amounts over a long period.

Drug Interactions: Antacids can interfere with the absorption of certain other medications. Therefore, a pharmacist should advise patients to take other medications 1 to 2 hours before or after taking an antacid.

Storage and Administration: Antacids should be stored at room temperature and out of reach of children. They should be chewed thoroughly before swallowing, and some may need to be taken with a full glass of water.

2. H2 Blockers

Histamine H2-receptor antagonists, also known as H2 blockers, are medications that decrease acid production in the stomach. They are commonly used to treat conditions that cause excess stomach acid, such as GERD.

Key points to cover in this section:

Mechanism of Action: H2 blockers work by blocking histamine from binding to H2 receptors on the stomach's parietal cells, which produce acid. By blocking these receptors, these medications reduce the production of stomach acid.

Common Types: Common over-the-counter H2 blockers include famotidine (Pepcid), cimetidine (Tagamet), and ranitidine (Zantac). Note: As of my knowledge cutoff in September 2021, ranitidine has been recalled worldwide due to potential contamination with N-nitrosodimethylamine (NDMA), a potential human carcinogen.

Usage: H2 blockers are used primarily to relieve GERD symptoms, prevent peptic ulcers, and treat gastric and duodenal ulcers. They are taken regularly, usually once or twice a day.

Side Effects: Common side effects include headaches, dizziness, diarrhea, constipation, and fatigue. In rare cases, they may cause confusion, especially in older adults.

Drug Interactions: H2 blockers can interact with certain medications, including anticoagulants, anti-seizure drugs, and certain heart medications. It's essential to discuss potential drug interactions with a healthcare provider.

Storage and Administration: H2 blockers should be stored at room temperature away from moisture and heat. They can be taken with or without food.

3. Proton Pump Inhibitors

Proton pump inhibitors (PPIs) are a type of medication used to reduce the production of stomach acid, and they are highly effective for treating GERD.

Key points to cover in this section:

Mechanism of Action: PPIs work by irreversibly blocking the enzyme system of gastric proton pumps, which are the final pathway for acid secretion in the stomach. This action significantly decreases stomach acid

production, providing more extended relief than antacids or H2 blockers.
Common Types: Over-the-counter PPIs include omeprazole (Prilosec), lansoprazole (Prevacid), and esomeprazole (Nexium).
Usage: PPIs are used for the treatment of frequent heartburn, GERD, gastric and duodenal ulcers, and erosive esophagitis. They are taken regularly, usually once a day, for a specified period.
Side Effects: Common side effects include headaches, nausea, diarrhea, abdominal pain, fatigue, and dizziness. Long-term use has been associated with an increased risk of bone fractures, vitamin B12 deficiency, and certain infections like Clostridium difficile.
Drug Interactions: PPIs can interact with certain other medications, such as clopidogrel (Plavix), certain antifungal drugs, and HIV medications. It's important to discuss potential drug interactions with a healthcare provider.
Storage and Administration: PPIs should be stored at room temperature and taken before meals, usually in the morning.

Review of Common OTC Products and Their Active Ingredients

There are three primary categories of OTC medications for treating GERD: Antacids, H2 blockers, and Proton Pump Inhibitors (PPIs). Here's a review of each category with some common product examples and their active ingredients:

1. **Antacids:**

   Tums: Calcium Carbonate
   Milk of Magnesia: Magnesium Hydroxide
   Maalox: Aluminum Hydroxide and Magnesium Hydroxide
   Alka-Seltzer: Sodium Bicarbonate and Aspirin
   Antacids work by neutralizing stomach acid, providing quick but temporary relief from heartburn and indigestion.

2. **H2 Blockers:**

   Tagamet (cimetidine): Cimetidine
   Pepcid (famotidine): Famotidine
   Zantac (ranitidine): Ranitidine (Note: As of my knowledge cutoff in September 2021, ranitidine has been recalled worldwide due to potential contamination with a probable human carcinogen.)
   H2 blockers work by reducing the production of stomach acid.

They provide longer-lasting relief than antacids but take longer to start working.

3. **Proton Pump Inhibitors (PPIs):**

   Prilosec (omeprazole): Omeprazole
   Prevacid (lansoprazole): Lansoprazole
   Nexium (esomeprazole): Esomeprazole
   PPIs work by blocking the enzyme system that produces stomach acid. They provide the longest-lasting relief but may take a day or more to start working.

IV. Patient Assessment and Recommendations
A. Asking the Right Questions:
When assessing a patient with GERD symptoms, it's important to ask the right questions to understand the frequency and severity of their symptoms, identify any potential triggers, and understand any other medications they may be taking that could interact with treatment options.

1. **Frequency:**
   How often do you experience these symptoms?
   Do you have symptoms at certain times of the day?
   Have you noticed an increase in the frequency of your symptoms?

2. **Severity:**
   How would you rate the severity of your symptoms on a scale of 1-10?
   Are your symptoms severe enough to interfere with your daily activities?
   Have you noticed any weight loss, difficulty swallowing, blood in your stool, or chest pain? (These could indicate a more serious condition and should be evaluated by a healthcare provider.)

3. **Triggers:**
   Have you noticed any specific foods, drinks, or activities that trigger your symptoms?
   Does your heartburn worsen after eating certain foods or lying down?
   Does stress or certain situations exacerbate your symptoms?

4. **Other Medications:**
   What other medications are you currently taking, including prescription drugs, over-the-counter medications, dietary supplements, or herbal remedies?

   Have you taken any over-the-counter treatments for your symptoms? If so, what have you taken and has it helped?

Based on the patient's responses, you can provide recommendations for over-the-counter treatments and lifestyle modifications. Remember, severe or persistent symptoms require evaluation by a healthcare professional, and any recommendation for an OTC product should be made with consideration of the patient's overall health status, potential drug interactions, and the safety and efficacy of the product.

B. Recommending Suitable OTC Products Based on Symptoms and Patient's Medical History

After conducting a thorough patient assessment, healthcare professionals can recommend suitable OTC products based on the patient's symptoms and medical history. Here are some general guidelines:

1. **Mild, Infrequent Symptoms:** If the patient experiences mild heartburn or acid reflux less than twice a week, an antacid like Tums or Mylanta could be sufficient. These provide rapid relief but are short-acting.
2. **Moderate, More Frequent Symptoms:** If the patient experiences symptoms more than twice a week, a H2 blocker like Pepcid or Tagamet may be more appropriate. These provide longer-lasting relief.
3. **Severe, Persistent Symptoms:** If the patient has severe symptoms that occur daily and interfere with daily activities, a proton pump inhibitor like Prilosec, Prevacid, or Nexium may be recommended. These medications offer the longest duration of relief but may take a day or more to begin working.

Consider the Patient's Medical History: Always consider the patient's medical history, including any known allergies, other medications they're taking, and any other health conditions they have. For example, antacids containing aluminum or magnesium should be used with caution in patients with kidney disease. H2 blockers and PPIs can interact with certain other medications, so ensure these won't interfere with any other treatments the patient is undergoing.

Lifestyle Modifications: In addition to OTC treatments, recommend lifestyle changes that can help manage GERD symptoms. This includes avoiding foods and drinks that trigger symptoms, eating smaller, more frequent meals, not eating within 2-3 hours of bedtime, elevating the head of the bed, and maintaining a healthy weight.

C. Providing Dietary and Lifestyle Advice: Foods to

Avoid, Weight Management, etc.

Dietary and lifestyle changes can play a significant role in managing GERD symptoms. Here are some general guidelines to provide to patients:

1. **Foods and Drinks to Avoid:** Certain foods and drinks can trigger GERD symptoms. Common triggers include:

    High-fat foods, Spicy foods, Citrus fruits and juices, Tomato-based foods, Chocolate, Mint, Coffee and other caffeinated drinks, Alcohol, and Carbonated beverages
    Patients should be encouraged to keep a food diary to identify personal triggers.

2. **Eating Habits:** Eating smaller, more frequent meals can help reduce GERD symptoms. Patients should also avoid eating within 2-3 hours of bedtime, as lying down after eating can contribute to acid reflux.
3. **Weight Management:** Being overweight or obese can put extra pressure on the stomach and increase the risk of GERD symptoms. If the patient is overweight, losing weight may help reduce symptoms.
4. **Physical Activity:** Regular physical activity can help with weight management and overall health, but certain exercises can worsen GERD symptoms. Avoid exercises that involve bending over or other movements that can increase abdominal pressure, such as certain yoga poses or weightlifting movements.
5. **Tobacco and Alcohol Use:** Both tobacco and alcohol can worsen GERD symptoms. Patients should be encouraged to quit smoking and limit alcohol consumption.
6. **Sleeping Position:** Elevating the head of the bed by about six inches can help prevent acid reflux during the night. Patients can do this using a foam wedge or by placing blocks under the head of the bed.

D. Recognizing When to Refer: Red Flags and Serious Symptoms

While OTC medications and lifestyle modifications can effectively manage mild to moderate GERD symptoms, it's crucial to recognize when a referral to a healthcare provider is necessary. Certain "red flags" or serious symptoms indicate the need for immediate medical attention:

1. **Persistent Symptoms:** If the patient's symptoms persist despite two weeks of treatment with OTC medications, they should be evaluated by a healthcare provider.
2. **Weight Loss:** Unintentional weight loss can be a sign of a serious condition, such as stomach or esophageal cancer.
3. **Difficulty Swallowing or Painful Swallowing:** These symptoms could indicate esophageal stricture or other serious conditions.
4. **Bleeding Symptoms:** Vomiting blood, black or tarry stools, or noticing blood in the stool can be signs of gastrointestinal bleeding, which requires immediate medical attention.
5. **Chest Pain:** While GERD can cause chest pain, it's important to rule out more serious conditions, such as heart disease. If the patient experiences chest pain, especially if it's accompanied by symptoms like shortness of breath, jaw or arm pain, or nausea, they should seek emergency medical care.
6. **Older Age:** Adults over the age of 50 with new-onset GERD symptoms should be evaluated by a healthcare provider, as the risk of esophageal cancer increases with age.
7. **Non-Responsive to Treatment:** If the patient's symptoms do not improve or worsen despite treatment, they should be referred to a healthcare provider.

Chapter Summary

This chapter focused on common digestive conditions such as constipation, diarrhea, and irritable bowel syndrome (IBS), emphasizing the importance of understanding the gastrointestinal tract and appropriate interventions.

:ints covered includeKey po

1. Constipation: Recognizing the causes, symptoms, and risk factors of constipation, and recommending the appropriate use of bulk-forming laxatives, stimulant laxatives, osmotic laxatives, and stool softeners.
2. Diarrhea: Differentiating between acute and chronic diarrhea, understanding causes such as infections or medication use, and advising on OTC treatments like loperamide and bismuth subsalicylate, alongside the importance of rehydration.
3. Irritable Bowel Syndrome (IBS): Understanding the symptoms of IBS and its impact on quality of life, while managing symptoms based on whether constipation or diarrhea is predominant, using fiber supplements, antidiarrheals, antispasmodics, and probiotics.

Practical Activity
A. Case Studies

Case Study 1:
A 35-year-old woman comes to the pharmacy complaining of constipation. She mentions that she has recently started a new job that is quite sedentary, and she's been eating a lot of fast food due to lack of time. She's otherwise healthy and takes no medications. She's looking for a quick fix to alleviate her discomfort.
Recommendation: This patient's lifestyle changes (sedentary job, fast food diet) could be contributing to her constipation. An OTC osmotic laxative like MiraLAX could provide short-term relief. In the long term, she should be advised to incorporate more fiber into her diet, drink plenty of water, and try to include more physical activity in her daily routine, even if it's just short walks during her break time.

Case Study 2:
A 75-year-old man is looking for a remedy for his constipation. He mentions that he usually has a bowel movement every other day, but for the past week, he hasn't been able to have one. He has a history of hypertension and takes a calcium channel blocker. He also mentions that he doesn't drink much water because he doesn't feel thirsty and worries about frequent urination.
Recommendation: The man's medication (calcium channel blocker) could be a contributing factor to his constipation. Also, his low fluid intake might be making his constipation worse. A bulk-forming laxative could be suitable, but given his age and medication use, it might be best to refer him to his healthcare provider to ensure there's no other underlying cause. In terms of lifestyle advice, he should be encouraged to increase his fluid intake, despite his concerns about urination.

Case Study 3:
Patient A is a 28-year-old woman who reports having frequent, loose stools for the past 3 days. She has no other symptoms and her medical history is unremarkable. She has been drinking water but has not tried any medications yet.
Recommendations: Acute diarrhea, likely due to a minor gastrointestinal bug or dietary trigger. No red flags or severe symptoms. Advise hydration and consider recommending an over-the-counter antidiarrheal, such as loperamide (Imodium). If symptoms persist beyond a few days or worsen, she should seek medical attention.

Case Study 4:

Patient B is a 35-year-old man who presents with symptoms of bloating and irregular bowel movements ranging from constipation to diarrhea for the past 6 months. He reports that his symptoms seem worse during periods of high stress at work.

Recommendations: These symptoms suggest IBS. The link between symptoms and stress suggests that stress management may be a key component of management.

Consider recommending a fiber supplement such as psyllium (Metamucil) to help regulate bowel movements and a probiotic to support gut health. Advise him to engage in regular exercise and stress management techniques. He should also consult with a healthcare provider to get a definitive diagnosis and further management.

Case Study 5:

Patient C is a 60-year-old woman who complains of diarrhea and abdominal pain for the past 2 weeks. She has lost weight and noticed blood in her stool a couple of times.

Recommendations: These are red flag symptoms, including prolonged diarrhea, abdominal pain, weight loss, and blood in the stool.

Recommend immediate medical attention. She needs a thorough evaluation by a healthcare professional to rule out serious conditions such as inflammatory bowel disease or colon cancer. OTC medications are not appropriate in this case without further medical evaluation.

Case Study 6:

Mr. Johnson, a 45-year-old man, walks into a pharmacy complaining of heartburn that he experiences about once a week, typically after eating spicy foods or drinking coffee. He's otherwise healthy and doesn't take any other medications.

Recommendation: Given the infrequency and trigger-based nature of Mr. Johnson's symptoms, an antacid like Tums or Mylanta, taken as needed after eating trigger foods, might be suitable for him. Additionally, he could be advised to limit his intake of spicy foods and coffee.

Case Study 7:

Mrs. Smith, a 55-year-old woman, complains of frequent heartburn that disrupts her sleep at night. She experiences this almost every day and antacids no longer provide relief. She's overweight and has a history of high blood pressure, for which she takes medication.

Recommendation: Given Mrs. Smith's frequent symptoms and the fact that antacids no longer provide relief, a proton pump inhibitor (PPI) like Prilosec might be a better fit. However, she should first consult her healthcare provider due to her high blood pressure and the fact that she's already on medication. Additionally, she may be advised to lose weight, avoid eating 2-3 hours before bedtime, and raise the head of her bed to manage her symptoms.

Case Study 8:
Mr. Davis, a 65-year-old man, complains of difficulty swallowing and weight loss, along with heartburn. He's a smoker and has been taking OTC Pepcid for the past three weeks with no relief.

Recommendation: Mr. Davis's symptoms are concerning, particularly the difficulty swallowing, weight loss, and lack of response to treatment. These could be signs of a more serious condition, such as esophageal cancer. He should be referred to a healthcare provider immediately. Furthermore, he should be advised to quit smoking, as this can exacerbate GERD symptoms and increase the risk of esophageal cancer.

B. Recommend OTC Products or Refer Based on Each Scenario

Scenario 1:
A 45-year-old woman comes to your pharmacy complaining of constipation. She says she's been under a lot of stress lately and hasn't been eating or exercising regularly. She doesn't take any regular medication and is generally in good health. She's looking for a short-term solution to get her back on track.

Scenario 2:
A 30-year-old man with irritable bowel syndrome (IBS) is experiencing a bout of constipation. He usually manages his condition with a combination of dietary changes and prescription medication, but he's been experiencing more constipation lately. He's looking for something he can take alongside his current treatment.

Scenario 3:
A 70-year-old man who recently had hip surgery is experiencing constipation. He's been taking a variety of pain medications since his surgery and thinks these might be causing his symptoms. He's looking for something safe he can take with his current medications to help relieve his constipation.

Scenario 4: A 28-year-old woman with frequent, loose stools for the past 3 days. No other symptoms and unremarkable medical history.

Scenario 5: A 35-year-old man with symptoms of bloating and irregular bowel movements ranging from constipation to diarrhea for the past 6 months. Symptoms worse during periods of high stress.

Scenario 6: A 60-year-old woman with diarrhea and abdominal pain for the past 2 weeks. She has lost weight and noticed blood in her stool a couple of times.

Scenario 7:

Mr. Thompson is a 30-year-old man who experiences heartburn about twice a week, usually after eating large meals. He's otherwise healthy and doesn't take any other medications.

Scenario 8:

Mrs. Rodriguez is a 50-year-old woman who complains of daily heartburn that sometimes wakes her up at night. Over-the-counter antacids provide some relief but not for long. She also takes medication for type 2 diabetes.

Scenario 9:

Mr. Lee, a 60-year-old man, complains of heartburn and a persistent cough. He's been taking OTC H2 blockers for a month with no relief. He's a smoker and occasionally drinks alcohol.

CHAPTER 4: SKIN CONDITIONS

I. Introduction
Overview of Skin Physiology and Function

1. **Protection:** The skin provides a physical barrier, protecting the body from mechanical impacts, pressure, temperature changes, micro-organisms, radiation, and chemicals.
2. **Regulation:** It plays a crucial role in body temperature regulation through sweating and changes in blood flow.
3. **Sensation:** The skin contains various types of nerve endings that respond to heat, cold, touch, pressure, vibration, and tissue injury, making it a sensory organ.
4. **Immune Response:** Langerhans cells in the skin are part of the immune system and help to detect foreign substances and defend against infections.
5. **Vitamin D Synthesis:** The skin is responsible for producing vitamin D when exposed to sunlight, which is essential for various bodily functions including the absorption of calcium.
6. **Excretion and Absorption:** Although not its main function, the skin does play a role in the excretion of toxins through sweat and the absorption of certain substances, like medication in the form of patches, through its layers.

II. Patient Assessment
A. Asking the Right Questions:

1. **Duration of the Condition:**

Understanding how long the patient has had the condition can help determine the seriousness and the need for further medical evaluation.
"When did you first notice the symptoms?"
"Has the condition been getting worse, better, or stayed the same?"

2. **Severity of the Condition:**
Knowing the severity of the condition can guide the selection of treatment and determine if a prescription medication might be necessary.
"How would you rate the severity of your symptoms on a scale from 1 to 10?"
"How much is the condition interfering with your daily activities?"

3. **Previous Treatments:**
Information about what treatments the patient has already tried can help avoid recommending something that was ineffective.
"Have you tried any treatments for this condition before? If so, what were they and how effective were they?"
"Did you experience any side effects from previous treatments?"

4. **Other Medications:**
Knowing what other medications the patient is taking can help avoid drug interactions.
"Are you currently taking any other medications, either prescription or over-the-counter?"
"Do you have any known allergies to medications?"

5. **Other Questions:**
"Are there any other symptoms accompanying your condition?"
"Have you been in close contact with anyone else with similar symptoms?"

B. Recognizing When to Refer: Persistent Symptoms, Severe Cases, etc.

Despite the efficacy of many over-the-counter (OTC) treatments, some cases will require a healthcare provider's attention. Knowing when to make this referral is an essential part of patient assessment. Here are some situations where a referral might be necessary:

1. **Persistent Symptoms:** If a patient has been using an OTC treatment as directed and their symptoms persist after several weeks, it may be time to refer them to a healthcare provider. Persistent symptoms could indicate a more severe or resistant condition that requires prescription treatment.

2. **Severe Cases:** If the patient's symptoms are severe.
3. **Systemic Symptoms:** If the patient is experiencing systemic symptoms, such as fever, joint pain, or fatigue in conjunction with their skin condition, this could indicate a more serious underlying condition and they should be referred to a healthcare provider promptly.
4. **Impact on Quality of Life:** If the condition is causing significant distress or impacting the patient's quality of life, it may be time to refer. This could include situations where the patient's sleep, work, or social interactions are being significantly affected.
5. **Uncertain Diagnosis:** If there's any uncertainty about the diagnosis - for example, if it's unclear patient's symptoms, a referral to a healthcare provider for a definitive diagnosis is needed.

Part 1: Hair loss

I. Introduction
Hair loss, or alopecia, is a common condition that affects millions of individuals worldwide, regardless of age or gender. It can manifest in various forms, ranging from thinning hair to complete baldness, and can result from a multitude of factors, including genetics, hormonal changes, medical conditions, and lifestyle choices.

Hair loss can be classified into several types, with androgenetic alopecia (male or female pattern baldness) being the most prevalent. Other types include alopecia areata, telogen effluvium, and traction alopecia, each with distinct causes and characteristics.

II. Understanding Hair loss
A. Definition and Symptoms
Definition: Hair loss, or alopecia, is a condition in which hair falls out in small patches, which can be unnoticeable. These patches may connect, however, and then become noticeable. The condition develops when the immune system attacks the hair follicles, resulting in hair loss.

Symptoms: Sudden hair loss that starts with one or more circular bald patches that may overlap.

B. Common Causes and Risk Factors
Causes: The exact cause of hair loss isn't well understood, but it's thought to be related to one or more factors including a family history of baldness, changes in the levels of male hormones (androgens), aging, and other factors.

Risk Factors: Age, family history, significant weight loss, certain medical conditions (like lupus and diabetes), stress, and some treatments like chemotherapy.

III. Over-the-Counter (OTC) Treatments
Topical Treatments for Hair Loss (Minoxidil)
Minoxidil is the only over-the-counter medication for hair loss approved by the FDA for use by both males and females. It belongs to a class of drugs known as vasodilators. It is not used for baldness at the front of the scalp or receding hairline in men. The foam and 2 percent minoxidil solution is also used to help hair growth in women with thinning hair. Minoxidil must be used indefinitely for continued support of existing hair

follicles and the maintenance of any experienced hair regrowth.
How to Use: It's typically applied to the scalp twice a day.
Side Effects: Side effects of minoxidil include irritation of the skin, itching, contact dermatitis, and dryness of the scalp or flaking.
Interactions: While minoxidil does not have many significant interactions, it's always important to check with a healthcare provider or pharmacist if it's being used in combination with other medications.

IV. Patient Recommendations
A. Recommending Suitable OTC Products Based on Symptoms and Patient's Medical History
When recommending over-the-counter (OTC) products, it's essential to consider both the patient's symptoms and their medical history. If the patient is experiencing gradual thinning or bald patches and has no known allergies or contraindications, a pharmacist might recommend an OTC product containing minoxidil, like Rogaine, which is appropriate for both men and women.

B. Providing Advice on Prevention and Hygiene Practices
Prevention and good hygiene practices are often the first line of defense against many common conditions. While genetic factors play a significant role in hair loss, certain practices can help prevent or slow it down. These include avoiding tight hairstyles that pull on the hair, avoiding harsh treatments like hot rollers, curling irons, and hot oil treatments, and eating a balanced diet that provides adequate protein, iron, and other nutrients essential for hair health.

C. Recognizing When to Refer: Persistent Symptoms, Severe Cases, etc.
Pharmacists play a vital role in the healthcare system by recognizing when a patient's condition requires a higher level of care. If the patient's hair loss is sudden, occurs in clumps, or is associated with redness, swelling, pain, or other skin problems, they should be referred to a healthcare provider. Additionally, if the hair loss continues or worsens after several months of using an OTC product like minoxidil, a referral is appropriate.

Part 2: Cold sores

I. Introduction
Cold sores, also known as fever blisters, are small, painful lesions that typically appear on or around the lips and mouth. They are caused by the herpes simplex virus (HSV), most commonly HSV-1, although HSV-2 can also be responsible in some cases. Cold sores are highly contagious and can be transmitted through close contact, such as kissing or sharing utensils.

Cold sores are one of the most prevalent viral infections worldwide, with a significant percentage of the population carrying the virus. Once infected, the virus remains dormant in the body and can reactivate due to various triggers, including stress, illness, hormonal changes, or sun exposure.

II. Understanding Cold Sores
A. Definition and Symptoms
Definition: Cold sores are small blisters that develop on the lips or around the mouth. They're caused by the herpes simplex virus and usually clear up without treatment within 7 to 10 days.

Symptoms: An itching, burning or tingling sensation around your mouth and on your lips before a blister appears. Each blister can contain several small fluid-filled sores which often join up before bursting.

B. Common Causes and Risk Factors
Causes: Cold sores are caused by the herpes simplex virus. There are two types of herpes simplex virus: HSV-1 and HSV-2. Both types can cause the symptoms of herpes, but HSV-1 is usually responsible for cold sores, and HSV-2 is most often the cause of genital herpes.

Risk Factors: Close personal contact with someone who has an active herpes infection, having a weakened immune system, exposure to UV light, hormonal changes, and stress.

III. Over-the-Counter (OTC) Treatments
Antiviral Creams for Cold Sores
These are topical antiviral medications used to treat herpes infections. When applied to the skin, they can speed up healing of the sores and decrease symptoms (pain, itching, burning, or tingling) in the early stages of a cold sore.

1. **Acyclovir (Zovirax):** Acyclovir cream is used to treat first outbreaks of genital herpes and to treat certain herpes simplex infections of the skin and mucous membranes.
   How to Use: It's typically applied to the affected area about five times per day for four days.
   Side Effects: Mild pain, burning, or stinging may occur. If these effects persist or worsen, tell your doctor or pharmacist promptly.
2. **Penciclovir (Denavir):** Penciclovir cream is used to treat cold sores on the lips and face caused by herpes simplex virus.
   How to Use: It's typically applied to the affected area every 2 hours while awake for four days.
   Side Effects: Mild pain may occur. If this effect persists or worsens, tell your doctor or pharmacist promptly.
   Interactions: While these topical antiviral creams do not have many significant interactions, it's always important to check with a healthcare provider or pharmacist if they're being used in combination with other medications.

IV. Patient Recommendations

A. Recommending Suitable OTC Products Based on Symptoms and Patient's Medical History

If a patient presents with a new cold sore, a pharmacist could recommend an OTC antiviral cream like Zovirax (acyclovir) or Denavir (penciclovir). The patient should start the treatment as soon as they notice the first symptoms for the best results.

B. Providing Advice on Prevention and Hygiene Practices

To prevent the spread of the virus that causes cold sores, avoid close contact (like kissing) with people who have active blisters. Don't share items that touch the mouth, such as lip balm, toothbrushes, and eating utensils. Using a lip balm with sunscreen may also help prevent cold sores triggered by sun exposure.

C. Recognizing When to Refer: Persistent Symptoms, Severe Cases, etc.

Patients should be referred if they have frequent outbreaks, if their sores are spreading or aren't healing after two weeks, or if they also have a fever, red eyes, sore throat, or other concerning symptoms. Patients with weakened immune systems should always be referred, as they are at higher risk of complications.

Part 3: Athlete's foot

I. Introduction
Athlete's foot, or tinea pedis, is a common fungal infection that primarily affects the skin on the feet, particularly between the toes. It is caused by dermatophytes, a group of fungi that thrive in warm, moist environments. Although it is commonly associated with athletes due to its prevalence in locker rooms and swimming pools, anyone can contract the infection.

Athlete's foot is highly contagious and can spread through direct contact with infected skin or surfaces. It is most often characterized by itching, burning, and peeling of the skin, especially in the web spaces between the toes.

II. Understanding Athlete's Foot
A. Definition and Symptoms
Definition: Athlete's foot is a fungal infection that usually begins between the toes. It commonly occurs in people whose feet have become very sweaty while confined within tightfitting shoes.

Symptoms: Itching, stinging, and burning between your toes or on soles of your feet, blisters that itch, cracking and peeling skin on your feet, most commonly between your toes and on your soles, dry skin on your soles or sides of your feet, raw skin on your feet, discolored, thick, and crumbly toenails.

B. Common Causes and Risk Factors
Causes: Athlete's foot is caused by a variety of fungal species that you can come into contact with when you walk barefoot in areas where someone else with athlete's foot has walked. Some people are simply more prone to this condition while others are resistant to it.

Risk Factors: Wearing damp socks and tight-fitting shoes, sharing socks, shoes, or towels with an infected person, walking barefoot in public areas where the infection can spread, such as locker rooms, saunas, swimming pools, communal baths, and showers.

III. Over-the-Counter (OTC) Treatments
Antifungal Treatments for Athlete's Foot
These are topical antifungal medications used to treat a variety of fungal infections, including athlete's foot. They work by stopping the growth of

fungi that cause infection.

1. **Terbinafine (Lamisil):**
   How to Use: Terbinafine cream or gel is typically applied once or twice daily for one to two weeks.
   Side Effects: Common side effects include irritation or itching at the site of application. If these effects persist or worsen, inform your doctor or pharmacist promptly.
2. **Clotrimazole (Lotrimin):**
   How to Use: Clotrimazole cream is typically applied to the affected area twice daily (morning and night) for 2 to 4 weeks.
   Side Effects: Skin irritation, burning, redness, and swelling may occur. If these effects persist or worsen, inform your doctor or pharmacist promptly.
   Interactions: While these topical antifungal creams do not have many significant interactions, it's always important to check with a healthcare provider or pharmacist if they're being used in combination with other medications.

IV. Patient Recommendations

A. Recommending Suitable OTC Products Based on Symptoms and Patient's Medical History

For a patient with itching, stinging, and burning on the feet, an OTC antifungal cream like Lamisil (terbinafine) or Lotrimin (clotrimazole) could be recommended. The choice between these may depend on the patient's past experiences with treatments, allergies, or any potential drug interactions with their current medications.

For all these conditions, it's crucial to advise the patient on how to use the product, what side effects they might experience, and when they should see improvements. If symptoms persist or worsen, patients should be advised to seek further medical attention.

B. Providing Advice on Prevention and Hygiene Practices

Good foot hygiene can help prevent athlete's foot. This includes washing feet daily with soap and water, thoroughly drying feet especially between the toes, changing socks regularly, and not sharing shoes. Wearing breathable footwear and using antifungal powders can also help prevent infection.

By providing advice on prevention and hygiene practices, pharmacists can help patients manage their conditions and prevent recurrence or worsening of symptoms.

C. Recognizing When to Refer: Persistent Symptoms, Severe Cases, etc.

If a patient's symptoms persist after two to four weeks of using an OTC antifungal treatment, they should be referred to a healthcare provider. Similarly, if they have severe cracking or scaling on the feet, signs of bacterial infection (like pus, redness, or swelling), or if they have diabetes, they should see a healthcare provider immediately.

In all cases, patients should be encouraged to seek medical attention if their symptoms worsen or persist despite self-care and OTC treatment, or if they develop new, unexplained symptoms. Pharmacists can help patients understand when their condition may require more specialized care.

Part 4: Dandruff

I. Introduction
Dandruff is a common scalp condition characterized by the shedding of dead skin cells, which can result in visible flakes on the scalp and shoulders. It often accompanies itching and irritation, and while it is not a serious health issue, it can be a source of embarrassment and distress for many individuals.

Dandruff affects a significant portion of the population, with both men and women experiencing it at some point in their lives. The condition can be classified into two main types: dry scalp dandruff, typically caused by dry skin, and seborrheic dermatitis, which is more severe and associated with oily skin and inflammation.

II. Understanding Dandruff
A. Definition and Symptoms
Definition: Dandruff is a common skin condition that primarily affects the scalp. It's characterized by the excessive shedding of dead skin cells from the scalp, leading to visible flakes in the hair and on clothing.

Symptoms: Common symptoms of dandruff include white or yellow flakes of skin on the scalp and hair, itching, and sometimes redness on the scalp.

B. Common Causes and Risk Factors
Causes: Dandruff can be caused by a variety of factors, including dry skin, sensitivity to hair products (contact dermatitis), and the overgrowth of a yeast-like fungus (malassezia) that lives on the scalp.

Risk Factors: Anyone can get dandruff, but certain factors can make you more susceptible. These include being male (men have larger oil-producing glands on their scalp), being of a certain age (young adulthood and middle age), having certain illnesses (such as HIV or Parkinson's disease), and having a diet lacking in certain types of vitamins.

III. Over-the-Counter (OTC) Treatments
Anti-Dandruff Shampoos

1. **Zinc Pyrithione Shampoos:** These are among the most widely used anti-dandruff shampoos. Zinc pyrithione is an antifungal

agent that reduces the amount of yeast on the scalp, a common cause of dandruff.
Example Products: Head & Shoulders, Selsun Blue Naturals, Dove Dermacare Scalp

2. **Selenium Sulfide Shampoos:** Selenium sulfide is another antifungal agent that can help reduce the presence of the Malassezia yeast on the scalp. It also helps to slow the death and shedding of skin cells on the scalp.
Example Products: Selsun Blue Medicated, Head & Shoulders Clinical Strength

3. **Ketoconazole Shampoos:** Ketoconazole is a potent antifungal medication that is very effective at reducing dandruff caused by yeast. It's available over the counter in lower concentrations and as a prescription in higher concentrations.
Example Products: Nizoral A-D

IV. Patient Recommendations

A. Recommending Suitable OTC Products Based on Symptoms and Patient's Medical History

When recommending an OTC product for dandruff, consider the severity of the patient's symptoms and their previous experiences with treatments. If they have mild dandruff and have not used any treatment before, a shampoo with zinc pyrithione, such as Head & Shoulders, could be an appropriate first option.

If the patient has tried zinc pyrithione shampoos without success, or if their symptoms are more severe, a shampoo with a stronger active ingredient like selenium sulfide or ketoconazole, such as Selsun Blue or Nizoral A-D, could be a good next step.

B. Providing Advice on Skin Care and Hygiene Practices

Whether the patient is dealing with dandruff or eczema, good skin care and hygiene practices can help manage symptoms and prevent flare-ups. Here are some general advice and tips:

1. **Regular Shampooing:** Regularly washing the hair with a gentle shampoo can help to reduce oil and skin cell buildup on the scalp, which can help to prevent dandruff.
2. **Proper Use of Anti-Dandruff Shampoos:** When using an anti-dandruff shampoo, it's important to massage it into the scalp and

leave it in for the recommended period of time before rinsing. This allows the active ingredients to work effectively.
3. **Diet and Hydration:** A balanced diet that includes enough zinc, B vitamins, and certain types of fats may help prevent dandruff. Also, staying well-hydrated can help maintain skin and scalp health.

Part 5: Eczema

I. Introduction
Eczema, also known as atopic dermatitis, is a chronic inflammatory skin condition characterized by itchy, red, and inflamed skin. It is one of the most common skin disorders, affecting individuals of all ages, particularly children. Eczema can significantly impact quality of life, leading to discomfort and emotional distress.

Eczema is often associated with other allergic conditions, such as asthma and hay fever. The exact cause is multifactorial, involving a combination of genetic, environmental, and immunological factors. Individuals with eczema typically have a compromised skin barrier, making their skin more susceptible to irritants and allergens.

II. Understanding Eczema
A. Definition and Symptoms
Definition: Eczema, also known as atopic dermatitis, is a chronic skin condition characterized by inflammation of the skin. It's most commonly seen in children but can occur at any age.

Symptoms: Eczema symptoms can vary widely but often include dry, red, itchy skin that can become cracked, swollen, and discolored. Eczema typically occurs in flare-ups, with periods of severe symptoms followed by periods of remission. It often affects areas like the hands, inner elbows, and the back of the knees, but it can occur on any part of the body.

B. Common Causes and Risk Factors
Causes: The exact cause of eczema is unknown, but it's thought to be linked to an overactive response by the body's immune system to an irritant. It is also believed to be related to a genetic variation that affects the skin's ability to provide protection from bacteria, irritants, and allergens.

Risk Factors: Eczema is common in families with a history of allergies or asthma, suggesting a genetic component to the disease. Other risk factors include stress, contact with irritants and allergens, and cold, dry climates.

III. Over-the-Counter (OTC) Treatments
Moisturizers and Topical Corticosteroids for Eczema

1. **Moisturizers:** One of the key elements in managing eczema is keeping the skin well-hydrated. Regular use of moisturizers can help maintain the skin's natural barrier, reduce dryness and itching, and potentially decrease the need for other medications. Moisturizers should be fragrance-free and hypoallergenic to avoid irritating the skin further.
   Example Products: Cetaphil, Eucerin, Aveeno Eczema Therapy, Vanicream
2. **Topical Corticosteroids:** These are anti-inflammatory medications that are used to reduce inflammation and itching. They come in various strengths, and the right one to use depends on the severity of the eczema, the age of the patient, and the location of the eczema on the body. Over-the-counter versions are milder, while stronger versions are available by prescription.
   Example Products: Hydrocortisone creams like Cortizone-10, Aveeno 1% Hydrocortisone Anti-Itch Cream

IV. Patient Recommendations
A. Recommending Suitable OTC Products Based on Symptoms and Patient's Medical History

1. **Mild to moderate eczema**: A regular moisturizing regimen with a product like Cetaphil or Eucerin can be beneficial. These moisturizers help to maintain the skin's natural barrier and reduce dryness, itching, and irritation.
2. **Eczema causing significant discomfort**: An OTC topical corticosteroid like hydrocortisone (Cortizone-10) could be recommended. This can help to reduce inflammation and itching. It's important to consider the patient's medical history when making these recommendations.
3. **History of allergic reactions to topical products**: Recommend products free from common irritants like fragrances.

B. Providing Advice on Skin Care and Hygiene Practices
Good skin care and hygiene practices can help manage symptoms and prevent flare-ups. Here are some general advice and tips:

1. **Moisturizing Regularly:** Keeping the skin moisturized can help to prevent dryness and reduce eczema symptoms. Use a thick, fragrance-free moisturizer immediately after bathing to lock in moisture.
2. **Avoid Triggers:** Eczema flare-ups can be triggered by a variety of factors, including harsh soaps, certain fabrics, fragrances, and allergens. Identifying and avoiding these triggers can help to prevent flare-ups.
3. **Brief, Lukewarm Baths or Showers:** Long, hot baths or showers can dry out the skin. It's better to take short baths or showers in lukewarm water.
4. **Gentle Skin Care Products:** Use skin care products that are hypoallergenic and free from irritants like artificial fragrances and dyes.
5. **Avoid Scratching:** Scratching can make eczema worse and lead to infection. Keep nails short and consider wearing gloves at night to prevent scratching.

Part 6: Warts

I. Introduction
Warts are benign growths on the skin caused by the human papillomavirus (HPV). They can appear anywhere on the body but are most commonly found on the hands, feet, and face. Though generally harmless, warts can be unsightly and may cause discomfort, leading individuals to seek treatment.

Warts are highly contagious and can spread through direct contact with an infected person or contaminated surfaces. There are several types of warts, including common warts, plantar warts, flat warts, and genital warts, each with distinct characteristics and locations.

II. Understanding Warts
Definition and Symptoms
Definition: Warts are small, fleshy bumps on the skin or the mucous membrane caused by infection with the human papillomavirus (HPV). There are several types of warts, including common warts, plantar warts, flat warts, and filiform warts.

Symptoms: Warts usually appear as a rough, grainy bump, often with a pattern of tiny black dots — these are small, clotted blood vessels. Depending on the type, they may occur on the hands, feet, face, or other parts of the body. Warts are usually painless, but some types, like plantar warts, can cause discomfort.

Common Causes and Risk Factors
Cause: Warts are caused by certain strains of the Human Papillomavirus (HPV). The virus is contagious and can spread through direct contact with a wart or with something that has touched a wart (like towels or razors).

Risk Factors: Anyone can develop warts, but some people are more susceptible. Risk factors include being a child or teenager (due to their less developed immune systems), having a weakened immune system (due to conditions like HIV or medications like immunosuppressants), and having a history of warts.

III. Over-the-Counter (OTC) Treatments
1. Salicylic Acid:

Description: Salicylic acid is a keratolytic (peeling agent) that causes shedding of the outer layer of skin. It's available in various forms, such as liquids, gels, and patches, and in different strengths.
How to Use: The acid is applied directly to the wart. Before application, soak the wart in warm water for about five minutes. After application, let the medication dry. Repeat this procedure once or twice daily as directed on the product packaging until the wart is gone (can take several weeks).
Considerations: Salicylic acid can irritate healthy skin around the wart. To protect the surrounding skin, apply petroleum jelly or a corn plaster around the wart. Avoid using salicylic acid on the face or genital area. It's not recommended for use on moles or birthmarks.

2. Cryotherapy:
Description: Cryotherapy involves freezing the wart using a very cold substance (usually liquid nitrogen). OTC cryotherapy products are available, often using a mixture of dimethyl ether and propane (DMEP).
How to Use: Follow the instructions on the product packaging. Typically, the product is applied directly to the wart. The freezing action causes a blister to form around the wart, and the dead tissue sloughs off within one to two weeks.
Considerations: Cryotherapy can cause mild to moderate pain, so it may not be suitable for everyone. It's also not recommended for use on the face or genital area. If the wart doesn't fall off after one treatment, you may need to repeat the process.

IV. Patient Recommendations
Recommending Suitable OTC Products Based on Symptoms and Patient's Medical History

When recommending OTC products, it's important to consider the patient's symptoms, the severity of the condition, their medical and treatment history, and any other medications they're currently taking.

1. **Small, non-painful wart**: An OTC salicylic acid product like *Compound W* or *Dr. Scholl's Clear Away Wart Remover* could be suitable. Remind the patient to protect the surrounding skin with petroleum jelly or a corn plaster.
2. **Larger wart or multiple warts and no contraindications**: An OTC freezing product like *Dr. Scholl's Freeze Away Wart Remover* could be an option.
3. **Warts on the face or genital area**: Recommend they see a healthcare provider instead of using OTC treatments.

Providing Advice on Prevention and Hygiene Practices

Educating patients about prevention and hygiene practices is an integral part of controlling the spread and recurrence of conditions like warts and scabies.

1. **Avoid Direct Contact:** Since warts are caused by a virus, they can be spread through direct contact. Avoid touching other people's warts or sharing personal items like towels or razors.
2. **Keep Skin Healthy and Unbroken:** Warts can invade the skin more easily if it's damaged or cut. Keeping the skin healthy and avoiding picking at warts can help prevent spread.
3. **Wear Protective Footwear:** To avoid plantar warts, wear flip-flops or pool shoes in public showers, locker rooms, and around public pools.

Recognizing When to Refer: Persistent Symptoms, Severe Cases, etc.

While many cases of warts and scabies can be treated with OTC products, some situations require referral to a healthcare provider for further evaluation and treatment.

1. **Persistent Warts:** If a wart doesn't improve after several weeks of OTC treatment or keeps returning, a healthcare provider should be consulted.
2. **Painful Warts:** Warts that are painful or bleed should be evaluated by a healthcare provider.
3. **Facial or Genital Warts:** Warts in these areas should always be evaluated by a healthcare provider due to the sensitive nature of the skin.
4. **Uncertain Diagnosis:** If the patient is unsure whether the growth is a wart, it's best to seek a professional opinion.

Part 7: Scabies

I. Introduction
Scabies is a highly contagious skin condition caused by an infestation of the Sarcoptes scabiei mite. This microscopic parasite burrows into the skin, leading to intense itching, irritation, and a characteristic rash. Scabies can affect anyone, regardless of age or hygiene, and is commonly spread in crowded conditions, such as nursing homes, schools, and shelters.

Scabies is transmitted through prolonged skin-to-skin contact with an infected individual or by sharing personal items, such as clothing or bedding. The mites can survive off the human body for a short period, making it important to treat both the infected person and their close contacts to prevent reinfestation.

II. Understanding Scabies
Definition and Symptoms
Definition: Scabies is a contagious skin condition caused by a tiny mite called Sarcoptes scabiei. The mites burrow into the upper layer of the skin where they live and lay eggs.

Symptoms: The primary symptom of scabies is intense itching, especially at night. Other symptoms include a pimple-like rash and sores caused by scratching. The burrows often appear as irregular track-like lines of tiny blisters or bumps on the skin. Common areas affected include between the fingers, wrists, elbows, armpits, waistline, and soles of the feet.

Common Causes and Risk Factors
Cause: Scabies is caused by the microscopic mite Sarcoptes scabiei. The mites burrow into the upper layer of the skin to live and lay eggs. Scabies is spread by direct, prolonged, skin-to-skin contact with a person who has scabies.

Risk Factors: Scabies can affect people of any age, race, and gender. However, you're at increased risk if you have close, prolonged contact with someone who has scabies, live in crowded conditions, or have a compromised immune system.

III. Over-the-Counter (OTC) Treatments
1. Permethrin Cream:

Description: Permethrin is a medication used to treat scabies. It's a synthetic pyrethroid that works by killing the mites and their eggs. It's often considered the treatment of choice for scabies.

How to Use: Permethrin cream (5%) is typically applied to the entire body from the neck down and left on for 8 to 14 hours before washing it off. The treatment may need to be repeated in a week if mites are still present.

Considerations: Permethrin is generally safe and effective. Side effects can include mild burning, stinging, or itching. Avoid contact with eyes, nose, and mouth.

2. Lindane Lotion:

Description: Lindane is an organochlorine insecticide also used to treat scabies. Due to its potential side effects, it's usually only recommended if other treatments have failed or can't be used.

How to Use: Lindane lotion is applied to the entire body from the neck down and washed off after 6-8 hours.

Considerations: Lindane can have serious side effects, including seizures and death, particularly when misused. It should not be used by pregnant or breastfeeding women, elderly, or individuals with a compromised immune system or skin conditions.

IV. Patient Recommendations
Recommending Suitable OTC Products Based on Symptoms and Patient's Medical History

1. **Scabies with no contraindications**: An OTC permethrin cream like *Nix* could be suitable. Remind the patient to apply the cream to the entire body from the neck down and leave it on for 8 to 14 hours before washing.
2. **Scabies resists permethrin, severe infestation, or permethrin contraindicated**: Recommend they see a healthcare provider for further evaluation. Lindane is another option, but due to its potential side effects, it's usually only prescribed when other treatments have failed or can't be used.

Providing Advice on Prevention and Hygiene Practices

Educating patients about prevention and hygiene practices is an integral part of controlling the spread and recurrence of conditions like warts and scabies.

1. **Immediate Treatment for Close Contacts:** Since scabies is highly contagious, it's recommended that all household members and other close contacts be treated at the same time, even if they're not showing symptoms.
2. **Clean Personal Items and Linens:** All clothing, bedding, and towels used by the infested person should be washed in hot water and dried in a hot dryer or sealed in a plastic bag for at least 72 hours.
3. **Avoid Close Contact:** Until successfully treated, avoid close physical contact and sharing personal items like clothing or bedding.

Recognizing When to Refer: Persistent Symptoms, Severe Cases, etc.

While many cases of warts and scabies can be treated with OTC products, some situations require referral to a healthcare provider for further evaluation and treatment.

1. **Persistent Symptoms:** If itching and rash persist for more than 2-4 weeks after treatment or the condition worsens, the patient should see a healthcare provider.
2. **Severe Infestation:** Cases with extensive skin lesions or severe itching may require stronger prescription treatments.
3. **Immunocompromised Patients:** Patients with a compromised immune system (due to conditions like HIV/AIDs or treatment with immunosuppressive drugs) should see a healthcare provider as they can develop a severe form of scabies known as Norwegian or crusted scabies.
4. **Infants, Young Children, and Pregnant or Nursing Women:** These individuals should be referred to a healthcare provider for treatment due to potential concerns with medication safety.

Chapter Summary

This chapter provided an overview of common skin conditions frequently encountered in community pharmacy practice, including their causes, symptoms, and available treatment options.

Key points covered include:

1. Hair Loss: Understanding the types and causes of hair loss (alopecia) and the role of treatments like minoxidil.
2. Cold Sores: Identifying the viral cause (herpes simplex) and recommending antiviral creams like acyclovir for symptom relief.
3. Athlete's Foot and Other Fungal Infections: Recognizing fungal skin infections like athlete's foot and treating them with topical antifungals such as clotrimazole or terbinafine.
4. Eczema and Dandruff: Managing inflammatory skin conditions with emollients, corticosteroid creams, and medicated shampoos for dandruff (seborrheic dermatitis).
5. Warts and Scabies: Differentiating between viral warts, often treated with salicylic acid, and scabies, a mite infestation treated with permethrin cream.
6. Patient Assessment: Asking the right questions to assess the severity of symptoms and choosing appropriate OTC products while identifying cases requiring medical referral.

Practical Activity
A. Case Studies

Case Study 1:
John, a 35-year-old man, approaches the pharmacy counter and mentions that he's been noticing more hair fall than usual when he showers. He's concerned about going bald, as his father started losing his hair at a similar age.
Recommendation: Ask John about his hair care routine, diet, stress levels, and any other symptoms. Assess if his hair loss is gradual or in patches.
If John's hair loss is gradual and resembles male pattern baldness, recommend an OTC product containing minoxidil, like Rogaine. Advise him on the application process and potential side effects.

Case Study 2:
Emma, a 28-year-old woman, comes into your pharmacy asking for something to help with a cold sore. She says it just appeared this morning and she has a big event in a week.
Recommendation: Ask Emma if she has had cold sores before and how often they occur. Also, inquire about her general health and any other medication she's taking.
Suggest Emma start treatment immediately with an OTC antiviral cream like Zovirax (acyclovir) or Denavir (penciclovir). Explain how to apply the cream and remind her to avoid close contact (like kissing) while she has an active blister.

Case Study 3:
Mike, a 42-year-old man, presents with itchy, red, and peeling skin between his toes. He says he recently started going to a new gym and noticed the symptoms a week ago.
Recommendation: Ask Mike about his foot hygiene habits and whether he's tried any treatments yet. Check if he has any health conditions like diabetes.
If Mike's symptoms align with athlete's foot without any severe signs, recommend an OTC antifungal cream like Lamisil (terbinafine) or Lotrimin (clotrimazole). Advise him on how to apply it and suggest some preventive measures like wearing flip-flops in communal showers at the gym.

Case Study 4:
A 35-year-old woman comes into the pharmacy complaining of a dry,

itchy scalp with visible flakes. She says she's been dealing with this issue for a few months, and it seems to worsen in the winter. She's tried a few different regular shampoos, but nothing has helped.

Recommendation: This patient's symptoms suggest she may be dealing with dandruff. Recommend an over-the-counter anti-dandruff shampoo such as Head & Shoulders, which contains the active ingredient pyrithione zinc and may help control her symptoms. She should use the product according to the instructions on the label, and if her symptoms persist after several weeks, or if they worsen at any point, she should seek medical attention.

Case Study 5:
A 22-year-old man comes in complaining of dry, itchy patches of skin on his hands and elbows. He's tried using a regular lotion, but it hasn't provided much relief. He also mentions the issue seems to be worse when he's stressed or when the weather is cold.

Recommendation: The symptoms described by the patient could be consistent with eczema. Recommend a moisturizing cream specifically formulated for eczema, such as Eucerin Eczema Relief Cream or Cetaphil Pro Eczema Soothing Moisturizer. If his symptoms are severe or causing significant distress, an OTC hydrocortisone cream like Cortizone-10 could provide additional relief. He should also try to identify and avoid potential triggers, such as stress and cold weather, and moisturize regularly. If his symptoms persist or worsen, he should seek medical attention.

Case Study 6:
A 35-year-old man comes to you with small, rough bumps on his hands, which he believes are warts. He's been treating them at home with an OTC salicylic acid product for two weeks but hasn't seen much improvement. He has no allergies or other health conditions.

Recommendation: The patient may need a stronger OTC treatment. Recommend trying an OTC freezing product like *Dr. Scholl's Freeze Away Wart Remover*. Remind him to follow the instructions on the product packaging and to seek medical attention if his condition worsens or doesn't improve after another two weeks of treatment.

Case Study 7:
A 50-year-old woman presents with an intensely itchy rash and small blisters on her wrists and between her fingers. She hasn't used any treatments yet. She has diabetes and is taking metformin.

Recommendation: The symptoms suggest scabies. An OTC permethrin cream like *Nix* could be suitable. Remind her to apply the cream to the entire body from the neck down and leave it on for 8 to 14 hours before washing. Also, instruct her to treat all household members and close contacts at the same time to prevent re-infestation. If her symptoms persist or worsen after two weeks, she should seek medical attention.

Case Study 8:
A 20-year-old college student comes to you with a painful wart on the sole of her foot. She tried an OTC salicylic acid product for a week, but the wart is still there.
Recommendation: She might benefit from an OTC freezing product like *Dr. Scholl's Freeze Away Wart Remover*. Remind her to protect the surrounding skin and to follow the instructions on the product packaging. If the wart doesn't improve or becomes more painful, she should see a healthcare provider.

Case Study 9:
A 28-year-old woman presents with symptoms of scabies but is pregnant. She has not used any treatments yet.
Recommendation: Given that she is pregnant, it's best to refer her to a healthcare provider. Some scabies treatments can be used in pregnancy, but this decision should be made by a healthcare provider who can weigh the benefits and risks.

Case Study 10:
A 45-year-old man comes to you with a small wart on his finger. He's previously tried a salicylic acid patch but saw no improvement after two weeks. He has no known allergies or other health conditions.
Recommendation: An OTC freezing product like *Dr. Scholl's Freeze Away Wart Remover* could be suitable. Remind him to follow the instructions on the product packaging and to seek medical attention if his condition worsens or doesn't improve after another two weeks of treatment.

Case Study 11:
A 16-year-old girl presents with intense itching and a rash on her torso, arms, and between her fingers. She believes she has scabies, as a friend she recently slept over with was just diagnosed. She has no known allergies but is asthmatic and uses an inhaler.
Recommendation: An OTC permethrin cream like *Nix* could be suitable. Remind her to apply the cream to the entire body from the neck down and leave it on for 8 to 14 hours before washing. Also, advise her to treat all household members and close contacts at the same time to prevent re-infestation. If her symptoms persist or worsen after two

weeks, she should seek medical attention.

B. Recommend OTC Products or Refer Based on Each Scenario

Scenario 1:
Susan, a 55-year-old woman, has noticed a significant increase in hair loss over the past two months. She says she's tried a variety of shampoos and hair treatments, but nothing seems to help. Susan also mentions that she has been under a lot of stress lately.

Scenario 2:
David, a 30-year-old man, comes to the pharmacy with a cold sore. He says it's his third outbreak this year. He has already tried an OTC antiviral cream, but the sores aren't improving.

Scenario 3:
Lisa, a 26-year-old woman, has been suffering from athlete's foot for over three weeks. She has been using an OTC antifungal cream consistently, but her symptoms haven't improved. The itching is severe, and she has begun to notice a foul smell.

Scenario 4:
Robert, a 68-year-old man with diabetes, asks for a recommendation for a rapid increase in hair loss over the past week. He hasn't tried any treatments yet.

For each scenario, consider the patient's symptoms, the duration and severity of their condition, their past treatments and current medications, and any other relevant factors in their medical history. Decide whether an OTC product might be suitable or if the patient should be referred to a healthcare provider. Remember to take into account the limitations of OTC treatments and the importance of early and appropriate medical intervention for certain conditions.

Scenario 5:
A woman experiencing a dry, itchy scalp with visible flakes.
Recommendation: An over-the-counter (OTC) anti-dandruff shampoo. Suitable options could include:
Head & Shoulders: Contains zinc pyrithione, which can help reduce dandruff.
Selsun Blue: Contains selenium sulfide, which can help control severe dandruff.

Scenario 6:
A man experiencing dry, itchy patches of skin on his hands and elbows.
Recommendation: An OTC product specifically designed for eczema. Suitable options could include:

Eucerin Eczema Relief Cream: This cream is specifically formulated for eczema and can help soothe dry, itchy, and inflamed skin.

Cortizone-10: If the patient's symptoms are severe, this OTC hydrocortisone cream can help reduce inflammation and itching.

In addition to recommending these products, advise the patient to try and identify potential triggers for his eczema flare-ups (such as stress and cold weather), and to take steps to avoid these triggers where possible. If his symptoms persist or worsen, he should be advised to seek medical attention.

CHAPTER 5: PEDIATRIC HEALTH

I. Introduction
Overview of Pediatric Pharmacology and Considerations

1. **Age and Development:** Children aren't just small adults - their bodies are continually growing and developing. These physiological changes can affect how children metabolize medications, often making them respond differently to drugs than adults.
2. **Dosing:** Determining the correct dose for a child isn't as simple as just scaling down an adult dose. It needs to take into account the child's weight, age, and sometimes surface area.
3. **Administration:** Pediatric patients may have difficulty swallowing tablets or capsules, so alternative forms, such as liquids or chewables, may be required. Taste can also be a significant factor in medication adherence in children.
4. **Safety:** Certain medications can be harmful or less effective in children. Pharmacists need to be aware of these and recommend alternatives when necessary.
5. **Communication:** Communicating with pediatric patients requires different strategies than with adults. Pharmacists should be skilled in explaining to children why and how to take their medication, and be able to reassure them and their parents or caregivers.
6. **Family-Centered Care:** Pediatric care often involves the whole family. Pharmacists should be prepared to answer questions from parents or caregivers and provide them with the necessary information to manage the child's condition at home.

II. Patient Assessment
Asking the Right Questions:
When assessing a patient and making recommendations, it's critical to gather information that can help determine the best course of action. Here are some key questions to ask:

1. **Duration of Symptoms**: *How long has the patient been experiencing symptoms?* Acute symptoms may indicate a different condition or require different treatment than chronic or recurring symptoms.
2. **Severity of Symptoms**: *How severe are the symptoms? Are they getting worse, staying the same, or improving?* This can help determine how aggressive treatment needs to be.
3. **Previous Treatments**: *What treatments has the patient already tried, if any? What was the result?* This can provide insight into what might work best for the patient moving forward.
4. **Other Medications**: *Is the patient taking any other medications, either prescription or over-the-counter?* This is critical to know in order to avoid any potential drug interactions.
5. **Allergies**: *Does the patient have any allergies to medications?*
6. **Underlying Conditions**: *Does the patient have any other health conditions that could be affecting their current issue or that could affect treatment?*
7. **Lifestyle Considerations**: *Are there any lifestyle factors that could be contributing to the condition or that could affect treatment?*

Part 1: Oral thrush

I. Understanding Oral thrush
A. Definition and Symptoms
Definition: Oral thrush, or oral candidiasis, is a condition where the fungus Candida albicans accumulates on the lining of the mouth. It's common in infants but can affect anyone.
Symptoms: Creamy white lesions on the tongue or inner cheeks, sometimes extending to the roof of the mouth, tonsils or back of the throat. In severe cases, it may spread into the esophagus, causing pain or difficulty swallowing.

B. Common Causes and Risk Factors
Causes: Caused by the overgrowth of the yeast Candida albicans in the mouth. The balance of bacteria and yeast in the mouth can be disrupted by illness, medications or stress, leading to oral thrush.
Risk Factors: Newborns, elderly people, and those with weakened immune systems are especially at risk. Other risk factors include use of corticosteroid inhalers, antibiotics, diabetes, and wearing dentures.

II. Over-the-Counter (OTC) Treatments
Antifungal Medications for Oral Thrush
Oral thrush is typically treated with antifungal medications. These can come in different forms, including lozenges, tablets, or liquids that you swish in your mouth and then swallow. While some antifungal medications may be available over-the-counter, others may require a prescription. It's important to consult a healthcare professional before starting treatment.

Here are a few commonly used OTC antifungal treatments for oral thrush:

1. **Nystatin oral suspension**: This is a liquid that is swished around the mouth and then swallowed or spit out. It is typically used 3-5 times a day for up to two weeks.
2. **Clotrimazole lozenges**: These are dissolved slowly in the mouth over 15-30 minutes, typically used five times a day for up to two weeks.
3. **Miconazole oral gel**: Applied in the mouth, it sticks to the mucosa, where it slowly releases the antifungal medication.

These medications work by killing the yeast that causes the infection. It's important to use the medication for as long as directed, even if the symptoms have improved, to ensure the infection is completely eliminated.

Part 2: Colic

I. Understanding the Colic
A. Definition and Symptoms
Definition: Colic is severe, often fluctuating pain in the abdomen that occurs in infants. While the exact cause is unknown, it's generally associated with the digestive system.
Symptoms: Infants with colic often cry or fuss for several hours a day, especially in the late afternoon or evening. Other signs may include clenched fists, arched back, or legs pulled up to the belly.

B. Common Causes and Risk Factors
Causes: The exact cause of colic is unknown. Some experts believe that colic is the result of an allergy, a change in the normal bacteria found in the gastrointestinal tract, a digestive disorder, or a combination of these.
Risk Factors: It appears in both first-born and later-born children, and affects boys and girls equally. Factors such as how a parent interprets a baby's crying or the anxiety level in the home can also influence the development of colic.

II. Over-the-Counter (OTC) Treatments
Treatment Strategies for Colic (Dietary Changes, Probiotics)
Colic is a challenging condition to manage as its exact cause is not known. However, there are several strategies that can help to soothe a colicky baby:

1. **Dietary Changes:** If you're breastfeeding, you might try eliminating dairy products, caffeine, onions, cabbage, and any other potentially irritating foods from your diet. If you're bottle-feeding, you might try a different brand or type of formula.
2. **Probiotics:** Probiotics, especially Lactobacillus reuteri, have been shown in some studies to reduce crying in some breastfed babies with colic. Probiotics can help restore the natural balance of bacteria in the baby's digestive tract.
3. **Over-the-counter remedies:** Some parents find that over-the-counter gas drops or gripe water (a mixture of water and various herbs) can help to reduce colic symptoms. However, the effectiveness of these treatments has not been proven.

4. **Feeding Changes:** Try feeding the baby more slowly, burping them more often during feedings, or moving to a bottle that limits the amount of air the baby swallows.

Part 3: Pinworm

I. Understanding Pinworm
A. Definition and Symptoms
Definition: Pinworm, or enterobiasis, is a common intestinal infection caused by tiny parasitic worms. It's most common in children.
Symptoms: The main symptom is itching in the anal area, particularly at night when the female worms lay their eggs. In girls, pinworm infection can also cause vaginal itching and irritation.

B. Common Causes and Risk Factors
Causes: The infection starts when a person ingests pinworm eggs. These eggs are usually spread by an infected person's dirty hands.
Risk Factors: Children and people living in crowded conditions, such as institutions, are most susceptible. The eggs can also be spread indirectly, in food, dust, or other items. The eggs can live on a surface for up to 3 weeks.

II. Over-the-Counter (OTC) Treatments
Pinworm infections are typically treated with over-the-counter or prescription anthelmintic (anti-parasitic) medications. These drugs kill the pinworms and help rid the body of the infection. Here are a few commonly used anthelmintic treatments for pinworm:

1. **Mebendazole (Vermox)**: This is a chewable tablet taken as a single dose, then repeated in two weeks. It's not recommended for children under 2 or pregnant women.
2. **Albendazole (Albenza)**: This is also a chewable tablet. Like mebendazole, it's taken as a single dose and repeated in two weeks.
3. **Pyrantel pamoate (Reese's Pinworm Medicine)**: This over-the-counter medication is taken as a single dose, then repeated in two weeks. It's safe for children as young as 2.

It's important to note that all members of a household should be treated with the medication, as pinworms are easily spread from person to person.
In addition to medication, good hygiene practices are critical for preventing the spread of pinworms. This includes washing hands

regularly, keeping fingernails short and clean, changing and washing underwear and bed linens frequently, and avoiding scratching the anal area.

Part 4: Napkin rash

I. Understanding the Napkin rash
A. Definition and Symptoms
Definition: Also known as diaper rash, it's a common form of inflamed skin (dermatitis) that appears as a patchwork of bright red skin on your baby's bottom. It's often related to wet or infrequently changed diapers, skin sensitivity, and chafing.

Symptoms: Skin signs include red, tender-looking skin in the diaper region — buttocks, thighs, and genitals.

B. Common Causes and Risk Factors
Causes: Diaper rash can be traced to a number of sources, including: Irritation from stool and urine, introduction of new foods, bacterial or yeast infection, and use of antibiotics.

Risk Factors: Infrequent diaper changes, chafing or rubbing, sensitive skin, use of antibiotics, and bouts of diarrhea can increase the risk of developing diaper rash.

II. Over-the-Counter (OTC) Treatments
Topical Creams and Ointments for Napkin Rash
Napkin (diaper) rash is a common problem in infants and toddlers, and can be managed effectively with over-the-counter (OTC) remedies. The key to treating diaper rash is to create a barrier that protects the skin from irritating substances and to keep the area as dry as possible. Here are some common types of OTC topical creams and ointments for napkin rash:

1. **Zinc Oxide Creams or Ointments**: These products, like Desitin or Balmex, create a protective barrier on the skin to shield it from moisture and irritants. They can be applied liberally and as often as needed with each diaper change, especially at bedtime when the diaper may be on for longer.
2. **Petroleum Jelly**: Products like Vaseline also create a barrier on the skin and can be used to prevent diaper rash or protect mild irritation.
3. **Hydrocortisone Creams**: Low-strength hydrocortisone creams can help calm inflammation and irritation. However, they should only be used for a short time and under a doctor's supervision.

4. **Antifungal Creams**: If the diaper rash is caused by a yeast infection, an over-the-counter antifungal cream like Lotrimin can be helpful.

Chapter Summary

This chapter focused on common pediatric conditions seen in community pharmacy, highlighting the pharmacist's role in offering safe and effective treatments for children.

Key points covered include:

1. Oral Thrush: Understanding the fungal infection (caused by Candida albicans) and recommending antifungal treatments like nystatin suspension.
2. Colic: Identifying the symptoms of colic in infants and advising on non-pharmacological approaches such as feeding adjustments and simethicone drops for gas relief.
3. Pinworm Infections: Recognizing pinworm infections and recommending appropriate treatments, such as mebendazole or pyrantel pamoate, along with hygiene advice to prevent reinfection.
4. Napkin (Diaper) Rash: Offering treatment advice on barrier creams (like zinc oxide) and antifungal creams for secondary infections, as well as prevention strategies like frequent diaper changes and keeping the area dry.
5. Safe Pediatric Dosing: Emphasizing the importance of accurate dosing for pediatric patients, especially with liquid medications, and educating caregivers on the use of dosing syringes or cups.

CHAPTER 6: MINOR EYE CONDITIONS

I. Introduction
Overview of Eye Anatomy and Physiology
Eye Anatomy:
The eye is a complex organ composed of many parts, each with a specific function:

1. **Cornea:** This is the clear, dome-shaped surface that covers the front of the eye. It helps focus light onto the retina.
2. **Iris:** This is the colored part of the eye. It controls the amount of light that enters the eye by changing the size of the pupil.
3. **Pupil:** This is the black circular opening in the center of the iris that allows light to enter the eye.
4. **Lens:** This is the clear part behind the iris, which helps focus light, or an image, onto the retina.
5. **Retina:** This is the light-sensitive tissue lining at the back of the eye. It detects light and converts it into signals which are sent through the optic nerve to the brain.
6. **Optic nerve:** This is the nerve that connects the eye to the brain. It carries the signals formed by the retina to the brain, which interprets them as images.
7. **Sclera:** This is the white part of the eye. It provides protection and form to the eye.
8. **Conjunctiva:** This is a thin, clear tissue that covers the front part of the eye and the inside of the eyelids.

Eye Physiology:
Eye physiology involves the functions of these parts to make vision possible:

1. **Light Refraction**: When light enters the eye, it is refracted, or bent, by the cornea and the lens to a point on the retina.
2. **Image Formation**: The retina converts the light into electrical signals. The retina's central area, known as the macula, is responsible for focusing central vision in the eye, and it controls our ability to read, drive a car, recognize faces or colors, and see objects in fine detail.
3. **Signal Transmission**: The optic nerve transmits these signals to the brain, which interprets them as visual images. The process is continuous and occurs in real time.

II. Patient Assessment and Recommendations
A. Asking the Right Questions:

When assessing a patient with a minor eye disorder, a structured approach can help determine the most appropriate advice and treatment recommendations. Here are some key questions to ask:

1. **Duration of Symptoms**: *How long has the patient been experiencing symptoms?* This can help differentiate between acute and chronic conditions.
2. **Severity of Symptoms**: *How severe are the symptoms? Are they getting worse or better?* Severe symptoms may necessitate referral to an eye care professional.
3. **Previous Treatments**: *Has the patient tried any treatments already? If so, what were they and what was the result?* This can provide insight into what has not worked and guide the next steps in treatment.
4. **Other Medications**: *Is the patient taking any other medications, either over-the-counter or prescription?* Certain medications can cause or worsen eye symptoms.
5. **Associated Symptoms**: *Are there any other symptoms associated with the eye disorder, such as a runny nose or fever?* This can help identify if the issue is part of a broader health problem.
6. **Contact Lens Use**: *Does the patient wear contact lenses?* Contact lens wearers may be at higher risk of certain eye conditions.
7. **Allergies**: *Does the patient have any known allergies, particularly to medications?* This is crucial information before recommending any treatment.
8. **Other Health Conditions**: *Does the patient have any other health conditions?* Certain conditions, like diabetes or autoimmune disorders, can affect eye health.

The answers to these questions can help determine whether an OTC treatment is appropriate or if the patient needs to be referred to an eye care professional. They can also guide the selection of the most suitable OTC product if one is deemed appropriate.

B. Providing Advice on Eye Care and Hygiene Practices

Proper eye care and hygiene practices can help prevent many common eye conditions and improve overall ocular health. Here are some tips to share with patients:

1. **Regular Hand Washing:** Hands should be washed thoroughly and frequently to avoid transferring dirt and bacteria to the eyes.
2. **Avoid Rubbing Eyes:** Rubbing the eyes can irritate them and may also introduce bacteria, leading to infections.
3. **Proper Contact Lens Care:** If a patient wears contact lenses, they should be instructed to clean and store them properly. This includes washing hands before handling lenses, using fresh solution every time lenses are stored, and replacing lenses as recommended by the eye care professional.
4. **Use of Protective Eyewear:** When engaging in activities that could potentially injure the eyes (like sports, woodworking, etc.), protective eyewear should be used.
5. **Limit Screen Time:** Prolonged digital screen use can cause eye strain and dryness. Patients should be advised to take regular breaks, follow the 20-20-20 rule (every 20 minutes, look at something 20 feet away for at least 20 seconds), and blink frequently.
6. **Eyelid Hygiene:** Regular cleaning of the eyelids with warm water or a recommended lid scrub can help prevent conditions like blepharitis.
7. **Regular Eye Check-ups:** Regular eye examinations can help detect eye conditions in their early stages when they are most treatable.
8. **Healthy Lifestyle:** A healthy diet rich in fruits and vegetables, particularly dark leafy greens and fish high in omega-3 fatty acids, can help maintain eye health. Regular exercise and not smoking can also benefit eye health.

C. Recognizing When to Refer: Persistent Symptoms, Severe Cases, etc.

Although many minor eye conditions can be managed with over-the-counter (OTC) products and proper hygiene practices, it's crucial to know when to refer a patient to an eye care professional. Some instances when referral is necessary include:

1. **Persistent Symptoms:** If a patient's symptoms persist despite using OTC treatments as directed, this could indicate a more severe or chronic condition that requires professional care.
2. **Severe Symptoms:** Symptoms like severe pain, intense redness, sensitivity to light, vision changes (like blurring or seeing spots), or signs of an eye infection (like yellow or green discharge) should be evaluated by an eye care professional promptly.
3. **Pre-existing Eye Conditions:** Patients with pre-existing eye conditions (like glaucoma, macular degeneration, or a history of eye surgeries) should be referred to an eye care professional for any new or worsening symptoms.
4. **Systemic Conditions:** Patients with systemic conditions that can affect the eyes (like diabetes, high blood pressure, or autoimmune diseases) should have regular check-ups with an eye care professional and should be referred if they experience any new eye symptoms.
5. **Trauma or Foreign Body:** Any trauma to the eye or the presence of a foreign body in the eye requires immediate professional care.
6. **Contact Lens Issues:** Contact lens wearers who experience discomfort, redness, or discharge should be referred, as these could be signs of a serious contact lens-related infection.

Part 1: Conjunctivitis

I. Understanding Conjunctivitis
A. Definition and Symptoms
Definition: Conjunctivitis **(Pink Eye)** is an inflammation or infection of the conjunctiva, the clear membrane that lines the eyelid and covers the white part of the eyeball. It can be caused by bacteria, viruses, allergies, or irritants like smoke or dust.

Symptoms: Redness in the white of the eye or inner eyelid, increased tear production, thick yellow discharge that crusts over the eyelashes, especially after sleep, green or white discharge from the eye, itchy or burning eyes, blurred vision, and increased sensitivity to light.

B. Causes and Risk Factors
Causes: Conjunctivitis can be caused by viruses, bacteria, allergens (e.g., pollen, dust mites, animal dander), irritants (e.g., smoke, pool chlorine, certain eye drops), and certain diseases that affect the whole body, like measles or the flu.

Risk Factors: Contact with someone infected with the viral or bacterial form of conjunctivitis, exposure to allergens or irritants, using contact lenses (especially extended-wear lenses), and having certain underlying diseases.

II. Over-the-Counter (OTC) Treatments
Antihistamines and Decongestants for Allergic Conjunctivitis

1. **Antihistamines**: These drugs work by blocking histamines, substances in the body that trigger allergy symptoms. Antihistamine eye drops can provide relief from symptoms of allergic conjunctivitis such as itching and redness. Examples include ketotifen fumarate (Zaditor, Alaway). Some oral antihistamines, like cetirizine (Zyrtec) or loratadine (Claritin), can also help reduce allergic reactions but may not be as effective for eye symptoms as eye drops.
2. **Decongestants**: Decongestant eye drops can help reduce eye redness associated with allergic conjunctivitis. They work by narrowing blood vessels in the eye to reduce redness. Examples include naphazoline (Clear Eyes Redness Relief) and

tetrahydrozoline (Visine). These should not be used for more than a few days at a time, as they could potentially exacerbate redness and irritation when overused (a condition known as rebound hyperemia).

Review of Common OTC Products and Their Active Ingredients

1. *Zaditor or Alaway*: These are antihistamine eye drops. The active ingredient in both products is ketotifen, which provides relief from itchy eyes due to allergies.
2. *Visine-A*: This is a combination of an antihistamine and a decongestant. The active ingredients are pheniramine maleate (an antihistamine) and naphazoline hydrochloride (a decongestant). This product can relieve itching and redness due to allergies.

Part 2: Dry eye syndrome

I. Understanding Dry eye syndrome
A. Definition and Symptoms
Definition: Dry eye syndrome is a condition in which a person doesn't have enough quality tears to lubricate and nourish the eye. It's often a part of the natural aging process, but it can also be caused by blinking or eyelid problems, medications, a dry climate, wind, and dust.

Symptoms: Stinging or burning eyes, stringy mucus in or around your eyes, sensitivity to light, redness of the eyes, a sensation of having something in your eyes, difficulty with nighttime driving, watery eyes (which is the body's response to the irritation of dry eyes), and blurred vision or eye fatigue.

B. Causes and Risk Factors
Causes: Dry eye syndrome can be caused by an imbalance in the tear mixture, insufficient tear production, or increased tear evaporation (often due to exposure to wind, smoke, or dry air). Certain medical conditions (like diabetes, thyroid disorders, and Vitamin A deficiency) and medications (like antihistamines, decongestants, hormone replacement therapy, and antidepressants) can also cause dry eyes.

Risk Factors: Aging (especially for post-menopausal women), long-term use of contact lenses, a diet low in vitamin A, and conditions that make it difficult to close the eye, such as Bell's palsy.

II. Over-the-Counter (OTC) Treatments
Artificial Tears and Lubricants for Dry Eye Syndrome
Artificial tears and lubricants are widely used as first-line treatments for dry eye syndrome. They provide symptomatic relief by supplementing the natural tear film and helping to moisturize the surface of the eye.

1. **Artificial Tears:** These are designed to mimic the content of real tears and to help supplement your body's natural tear production. They can provide temporary relief from burning and irritation related to dry eye syndrome. Examples of artificial tears include brands such as Systane, Refresh, and TheraTears. Some contain preservatives to prolong shelf life, while others are preservative-free for those who are sensitive or who need to use drops frequently.

2. **Lubricating Eye Ointments**: These are thicker than artificial tears and provide longer-lasting relief for dry eyes, especially during the night. They can cause temporary blurred vision and are typically recommended for use before bedtime. Examples include brands like Systane Nighttime and Refresh PM.
3. **Lubricating Eye Gels**: These products provide a thicker layer of protection than regular artificial tears but are less thick than ointments. They offer longer relief and can be used less frequently than artificial tears. An example is Systane Gel Drops.

Review of Common OTC Products and Their Active Ingredients

1. *Systane Balance*: This is a lubricant eye drop. The active ingredients are propylene glycol and hydroxypropyl guar. These ingredients work together to provide instant relief and extended protection against dry eye symptoms.
2. *Refresh Tears*: This is a lubricant eye drop. The active ingredient is carboxymethylcellulose sodium, which provides immediate, soothing relief for dry, irritated eyes.
3. *TheraTears*: This is a lubricant eye drop. The active ingredient is sodium carboxymethylcellulose, which helps to restore, cleanse, and nourish the eyes.

Part 3: Blepharitis

I. Understanding Blepharitis
A. Definition and Symptoms
Definition: Blepharitis is an inflammation of the eyelids, usually where the eyelashes grow, causing red, irritated, itchy eyelids and the formation of dandruff-like scales on eyelashes.
Symptoms: Red, swollen eyelids, a burning or stinging eye, crusty debris or dandruff at the base of eyelashes, a gritty or sandy sensation in the eye, itchy eyelids, and frequent blinking.

B. Causes and Risk Factors
Causes: Blepharitis is often associated with a bacterial infection, skin conditions (like seborrheic dermatitis or acne rosacea), malfunctioning oil glands in the eyelid, or allergic reactions.
Risk Factors: Having dandruff or oily skin, a history of allergic reactions, eyelash lice or mites, and certain systemic conditions like rosacea.

II. Over-the-Counter (OTC) Treatments
Eyelid Cleansing Products for Blepharitis
Good eyelid hygiene is the cornerstone of managing blepharitis. Over-the-counter eyelid cleansing products can help reduce symptoms and prevent further episodes. These products typically come in the form of solutions, wipes, or foams, and are designed to remove excess oils, debris, and other irritants that can contribute to inflammation.

1. **Eyelid Cleansing Solutions:** These are liquids used to clean the eyelids and lashes. They often contain ingredients designed to break down and remove oil and debris. Examples include OCuSOFT Lid Scrub Plus and Heyedrate Lid and Lash Cleanser.
2. **Eyelid Cleansing Wipes:** These are pre-moistened pads or wipes that are used to clean the eyelid area. They are convenient and portable. Examples include Systane Lid Wipes and Blephaclean Eyelid Cleansing Wipes.
3. **Eyelid Cleansing Foams:** These are foaming cleansers applied to the eyelids and then rinsed off. They can provide a deep clean and are often recommended for more severe or persistent cases

of blepharitis. An example is OCuSOFT Lid Scrub Foaming Eyelid Cleanser.

Review of Common OTC Products and Their Active Ingredients

1. *OCuSOFT Lid Scrub Plus*: This is an eyelid cleanser. The active ingredient is cocamidopropyl betaine, which effectively removes oil and debris from the eyelids.
2. *Systane Lid Wipes*: These are pre-moistened eyelid cleansing wipes. They do not contain any medication, but they effectively remove oil and debris from the eyelids.
3. *Heyedrate Lid and Lash Cleanser*: This is a hypochlorous acid eyelid and lash cleanser. The active ingredient is pure hypochlorous acid, which cleanses the eyelids and promotes overall eye health.

Practical Activity
A. Case Studies
Case Study 1:
Patient A is a 30-year-old woman who complains of itchy, red eyes. She reports that she started experiencing these symptoms a week ago, and they seem to get worse when she's outside. She has tried using artificial tears, but they don't seem to help. The patient also mentions that she suffers from seasonal allergies.

Recommendation: The patient's symptoms and history of seasonal allergies suggest that she may be experiencing allergic conjunctivitis. An OTC antihistamine eye drop like Zaditor or Alaway could be recommended. If symptoms persist or worsen, she should be advised to see an eye care professional.

Case Study 2:
Patient B is a 45-year-old man who has been experiencing dry, gritty-feeling eyes for several months. He works as a software developer and spends a lot of time in front of a computer screen. The patient has tried using artificial tears a few times a day, but his symptoms still persist.

Recommendation: Patient B's symptoms and job suggest that he might be experiencing dry eye syndrome, possibly exacerbated by prolonged screen time. He could benefit from frequent use of lubricant eye drops such as Systane or Refresh Tears, and possibly a gel or ointment at night for more prolonged relief. Additionally, advising him on the importance of regular breaks from the screen, blinking exercises, and maintaining a healthy indoor environment (avoiding dry air) could help. If symptoms persist, he should be referred to an eye care professional for further evaluation and treatment.

B. Recommend OTC Products or Refer Based on Each Scenario
Scenario 1:
Patient C is a 60-year-old woman who complains of burning and stinging eyes for the past week. She also mentions that she has a rheumatic condition and takes several medications for it. She hasn't tried any eye drops yet.

Scenario 2:
Patient D is a 20-year-old college student who complains of red, itchy eyes with a yellowish discharge that started three days ago. He wears contact lenses and admits that he doesn't always clean them properly. He tried using his friend's antibiotic eye drops, but his symptoms have worsened.

Note: Take into account the patient's symptoms, their duration, severity, response to any previous treatments, their overall medical history, and lifestyle context. Remember the importance of recognizing when to recommend an OTC treatment and when to refer the patient to an eye care professional.

Differences between Conditions

The differences between these minor eye disorders - conjunctivitis, dry eye syndrome, and blepharitis - lie mainly in their causes, symptoms, and treatment approaches:

1. Conjunctivitis:

Cause: Often caused by a bacterial or viral infection, an allergic reaction, or an irritant like smoke or dust.

Symptoms: Symptoms include redness, itching, and a discharge that can be clear, white, yellow, or green. The eyes may also feel gritty and may water more than usual.

Treatment: Depending on the cause, treatment may involve antibiotic eye drops or ointments for bacterial conjunctivitis, antihistamines for allergic conjunctivitis, or simply avoiding the irritant. Viral conjunctivitis usually resolves on its own without treatment.

2. Dry Eye Syndrome:

Cause: Dry eye syndrome occurs when the eye does not produce tears properly, or when the tears are not of the correct consistency and evaporate too quickly.

Symptoms: Symptoms include stinging or burning of the eye, a sandy or gritty feeling as if something is in the eye, episodes of excess tears following very dry eye periods, and discomfort when reading, working on a computer, or being in a dry environment.

Treatment: Treatment often involves over-the-counter eye drops or prescription medications to stimulate tear production, as well as lifestyle changes like taking breaks during computer work, avoiding wind and dry air, and using a humidifier.

3. Blepharitis:

Cause: Blepharitis is usually caused by an overgrowth of the bacteria that live along the margins of the eyelids, although it can also be associated with skin conditions such as rosacea and dandruff.

Symptoms: Symptoms include red and swollen eyelids, crusty eyelashes (especially upon waking), itchy eyes, a burning sensation, and occasionally blurred vision.

Treatment: Treatment often involves good eyelid hygiene such as regular cleaning and warm compresses, as well as antibiotic ointments in some cases.

Chapter Summary

In this chapter, we explored common minor eye disorders that pharmacists frequently manage, with an emphasis on understanding symptoms, causes, and suitable over-the-counter treatments.

Key points covered include:

1. Conjunctivitis: Differentiating between bacterial, viral, and allergic conjunctivitis, and recommending treatments such as lubricating eye drops for viral/allergic conjunctivitis or antibiotic eye drops for bacterial cases.
2. Dry Eye Syndrome: Identifying the causes of dry eyes, such as environmental factors or prolonged screen use, and advising on artificial tears and lubricating eye drops for symptom relief.
3. Blepharitis: Understanding this chronic inflammation of the eyelids and suggesting treatments like lid hygiene (warm compresses) and gentle cleansing with lid wipes or diluted baby shampoo.
4. Patient Assessment: Asking the right questions to assess eye symptoms, their duration, and any associated conditions, and determining when to refer patients for further medical evaluation, particularly in cases of vision loss or severe pain.

CHAPTER 7: WOMEN'S HEALTH

I. Introduction
Overview of Key Aspects of Women's Health

1. **Menstrual Health**: This involves understanding the normal menstrual cycle, common disorders such as premenstrual syndrome (PMS), dysmenorrhea, and amenorrhea, and the impact of menstrual health on overall wellbeing.
2. **Reproductive Health**: This includes topics like contraception, sexually transmitted infections (STIs), fertility, pregnancy, and menopause.
3. **Breast Health**: Understanding the importance of regular self-examinations, awareness of changes, and mammograms for early detection of breast cancer.
4. **Bone Health**: Emphasizing the importance of maintaining bone density, understanding the increased risk of osteoporosis in postmenopausal women, and the role of diet, exercise, and supplements in prevention.
5. **Urinary Health**: Awareness of urinary tract infections (UTIs), which are more common in women due to anatomical differences, and the importance of hydration and hygiene.
6. **Mental Health**: Recognition of the impact of hormonal changes on mood and mental wellbeing, and the importance of addressing mental health issues such as depression, anxiety, and postpartum depression.
7. **Cardiovascular Health**: Understanding that heart disease is a leading cause of death for women and awareness of the unique symptoms of heart disease in women.

8. **Preventive Care and Screenings**: Importance of regular check-ups, pap smears, and other screenings for early detection and prevention of diseases.

II. Patient Assessment
Asking the Right Questions:

1. **Understanding the Patient's Symptoms**: Ask about the nature of their symptoms - what they are, when they started, how severe they are, if anything makes them better or worse, and if they've tried any treatments. For example, if a patient complains of a headache, ask about the type of pain, its location, duration, triggers, and any associated symptoms.
2. **Medical History**: Inquire about any diagnosed medical conditions, past surgeries or hospitalizations, allergies, and lifestyle habits (smoking, alcohol, diet, exercise). This information can help identify potential causes of symptoms or contraindications to certain OTC treatments.
3. **Current Medications**: Ask about both prescription and over-the-counter medications, as well as any supplements or herbal products the patient may be taking. This can help identify potential drug interactions or side effects that may be contributing to their symptoms.

After gathering this information, the pharmacist can make a recommendation. This might include suggesting an OTC product, providing lifestyle advice, or referring the patient to a doctor if their symptoms suggest a more serious condition that requires medical evaluation.

Part 1: Menstrual disorders

I. Understanding Menstrual disorders
A. Definitions

1. **Premenstrual Syndrome (PMS)**: A group of symptoms that occur a week or two before menstruation. Symptoms can be physical (bloating, breast tenderness, headaches) and emotional (mood swings, irritability, depression).
2. **Dysmenorrhea**: Painful menstruation that can interfere with daily activities. Primary dysmenorrhea is due to the menstrual process itself, while secondary dysmenorrhea is caused by another medical condition, like endometriosis.
3. **Menorrhagia (heavy periods)**: Menstrual bleeding that lasts more than 7 days or is excessively heavy. It can lead to anemia if not managed properly.
4. **Amenorrhea**: The absence of menstrual periods. Primary amenorrhea is when menstruation hasn't begun by age 16. Secondary amenorrhea is when previously regular periods stop for at least 3 months.

B. Symptoms and Risk Factors
Symptoms: Abnormal bleeding, heavy periods, painful cramps, bloating, irritability, mood swings, absence of periods.
Risk Factors: Age, family history, obesity, stress, smoking, and certain medical conditions like polycystic ovary syndrome (PCOS) or endometriosis.

C. Importance of Early Detection and Management
Early detection of abnormal menstrual patterns can help diagnose underlying conditions like polycystic ovary syndrome (PCOS), endometriosis, or even reproductive organ cancers. Early management can reduce discomfort, prevent complications like anemia, and improve a woman's overall quality of life.

II. Over-the-Counter (OTC) Treatments and Prescription Medications
Non-prescription Options:
Nonsteroidal anti-inflammatory drugs (NSAIDs), like ibuprofen or

naproxen, can be recommended for pain and inflammation. Heat patches or warm baths can also help relieve discomfort.

Review of Common OTC Products and Their Active Ingredients Pain Relief for Menstrual Discomfort:

1. Ibuprofen (Advil, Motrin)
2. Naproxen Sodium (Aleve)
3. Acetaminophen (Tylenol)

III. Patient Recommendations
A. Recommending Suitable OTC Products or Referring for Physician Consultation

For mild to moderate pain, recommend NSAIDs like ibuprofen or naproxen. If symptoms are severe, persistent, or accompanied by other worrying signs such as heavy bleeding or irregular periods, refer the patient to a healthcare provider for further evaluation.

B. Providing Advice on Lifestyle Modifications and Preventative Health Measures

Encourage a healthy diet and regular exercise, which can sometimes help regulate menstrual cycles. For those with severe pain, relaxation techniques and heat therapy can be beneficial.

Part 2: Urinary Tract Infections (UTI)

I. Understanding UTI
A. Definition
Common infections that occur when bacteria enter the urinary tract. Symptoms can include a frequent urge to urinate, pain or burning during urination, and cloudy urine. UTIs are more common in women due to anatomical differences.

B. Symptoms and Risk Factors for Each Condition
Symptoms: Frequent urge to urinate, discomfort or burning sensation during urination, lower abdominal pain, cloudy or strong-smelling urine, fever (in more severe cases).
Risk Factors: Female anatomy (a shorter urethra), sexual activity, certain types of birth control (like diaphragms), menopause (due to a decrease in protective vaginal bacteria), and conditions that obstruct urine flow (like kidney stones).

C. Importance of Early Detection and Management
Early detection and treatment of UTIs can prevent the spread of infection to the kidneys, which can lead to more severe health problems. Effective management includes appropriate antibiotic use and advice on prevention strategies.

II. Over-the-Counter (OTC) Treatments and Prescription Medications
A. Non-prescription Options
While antibiotics are needed to treat UTIs, over-the-counter urinary pain relief medication (phenazopyridine) can be used to relieve symptoms. Encourage hydration and the use of urinary alkalinizers to help ease discomfort.

B. Prescription Medications
Antibiotics:
Antibiotics are used for treating urinary tract infections (UTIs). The choice of antibiotic depends on the specific bacteria causing the infection, patient allergies, and other factors.
It's essential to educate patients about the importance of taking the full course of antibiotics, even if they feel better, to prevent antibiotic

resistance.

Review of Common OTC Products and Their Active Ingredients

1. Phenazopyridine Hydrochloride (Azo Urinary Pain Relief)
2. Sodium bicarbonate/citric acid (urinary alkalinizers like Ural)

III. Patient Recommendations
A. Recommending Suitable OTC Products or Referring for Physician Consultation

UTIs should be treated by a healthcare provider because they require antibiotics, which are not available over the counter. However, for immediate relief of symptoms, you can recommend phenazopyridine. Always refer the patient to a physician for an appropriate antibiotic prescription.

B. Providing Advice on Lifestyle Modifications and Preventative Health Measures

Advise patients to drink plenty of fluids and urinate regularly, especially after sexual intercourse. Also, recommend proper hygiene practices to prevent bacteria from entering the urinary tract.

Part 3: Menopause

I. Understanding Menopause
A. Definition
A natural biological process marking the end of menstrual cycles. It's diagnosed after going 12 months without a menstrual period. Symptoms can include hot flashes, night sweats, sleep problems, and mood changes. Long-term effects can include osteoporosis and heart disease.

B. Symptoms and Risk Factors
Symptoms: Irregular periods, hot flashes, night sweats, sleep disturbances, mood changes, dry skin and mucous membranes, decreased breast fullness.
Risk Factors: Age is the primary factor, but early menopause can be induced by certain medical treatments, or it may be genetic. Smoking can also lead to early menopause.

C. Importance of Early Detection and Management
Detecting the onset of menopause can help manage its symptoms and mitigate related health risks like osteoporosis and heart disease. Early management might include lifestyle modifications, hormone replacement therapy, or other symptomatic treatments.

II. Over-the-Counter (OTC) Treatments and Prescription Medications
A. Non-prescription Options
Over-the-counter treatments can include phytoestrogens (like soy and red clover), black cohosh for hot flashes, and vaginal moisturizers for dryness. Always remind patients to discuss these options with their healthcare provider as they can interfere with other medications or conditions.

B. Prescription Medications
Hormone Therapy:
Used primarily to treat symptoms of menopause, such as hot flashes and vaginal dryness. They can also protect against osteoporosis. Hormone therapy can come in systemic products, which treat widespread symptoms, or local products that treat only specific symptoms.

There are risks associated with hormone therapy, such as blood clots, heart disease, and certain cancers, so it's essential to use the lowest effective dose for the shortest time needed.

Review of Common OTC Products and Their Active Ingredients

1. Black Cohosh (Remifemin, MenoEase360)
2. Soy Isoflavones (various brands)

III. Patient Recommendations
A. Recommending Suitable OTC Products or Referring for Physician Consultation

For mild menopausal symptoms, suggest over-the-counter remedies like black cohosh for hot flashes or non-hormonal vaginal moisturizers for dryness. If symptoms are severe or significantly affecting the patient's quality of life, referral to a healthcare provider for potential hormone replacement therapy may be appropriate.

B. Providing Advice on Lifestyle Modifications and Preventative Health Measures

Suggest lifestyle changes that can help manage symptoms. These can include maintaining a cool environment, wearing light clothing, and avoiding triggers for hot flashes like spicy foods and caffeine. Regular exercise can also help manage symptoms and improve overall health.

Part 4: Osteoporosis

I. Understanding Osteoporosis
A. Definition
A bone disease that occurs when the body loses too much bone, makes too little bone, or both. As a result, bones become weak and may break from a fall or, in severe cases, from minor bumps. It's more common in postmenopausal women due to lower estrogen levels.

B. Symptoms and Risk Factors
Symptoms: Often no symptoms until a fracture occurs. In severe cases, a stooped posture, back pain, and loss of height over time can occur.
Risk Factors: Age, being female, menopause, family history, low body weight, use of certain medications (like corticosteroids), certain diseases (like rheumatoid arthritis), and lifestyle factors (smoking, excessive alcohol, lack of physical activity).

C. Importance of Early Detection and Management
Early detection, often through bone density testing, is crucial in preventing osteoporosis-related fractures, which can lead to chronic pain, disability, loss of independence, or even death. Management strategies include medication, adequate intake of calcium and vitamin D, and regular weight-bearing exercise.

II. Over-the-Counter (OTC) Treatments and Prescription Medications
A. Non-prescription Options
Calcium and Vitamin D supplements are generally recommended to help maintain bone health. Weight-bearing exercises are also important for bone health.

B. Prescription Medications
Bisphosphonates:
Bisphosphonates are a type of medication used to slow bone loss, increase bone density, and reduce the risk of broken bones in people with osteoporosis.
Side effects can include digestive problems and, very rarely, damage to the jawbone or atypical femur fractures.
They are typically taken once a week or once a month, and it's crucial to

take them correctly to maximize absorption and minimize side effects.

C. Review of Common OTC Products and Their Active Ingredients
Bone Health:

1. Calcium (Caltrate, Tums)
2. Vitamin D3 (Ddrops, Nature's Bounty Vitamin D3)

III. Patient Recommendations
A. Recommending Suitable OTC Products or Referring for Physician Consultation

Recommend calcium and vitamin D supplements to help maintain bone health. However, if the patient has been diagnosed with osteoporosis or has significant risk factors (like a family history, being postmenopausal, or having a low body weight), referral to a healthcare provider is necessary for potential prescription medication.

B. Providing Advice on Lifestyle Modifications and Preventative Health Measures

Advocate for a diet rich in calcium and vitamin D, regular weight-bearing exercise (like walking or weightlifting), and avoiding smoking and excessive alcohol, which can decrease bone density.

Good lifestyle choices can often prevent or manage many health conditions. It's important to remind patients that these suggestions should complement, not replace, traditional medical treatments. It's also essential to individualize advice based on the patient's current lifestyle, preferences, and overall health status.

Chapter Summary

This chapter covered common women's health issues that pharmacists frequently manage, focusing on the treatment of menstrual, urinary, and hormonal conditions.

Key points covered include:

1. Menstrual Disorders: Understanding conditions like dysmenorrhea (painful periods) and recommending OTC treatments such as NSAIDs (ibuprofen) for pain relief, along with lifestyle advice to manage symptoms.
2. Urinary Tract Infections (UTIs): Recognizing the symptoms of UTIs, including frequent urination and burning, and advising on the use of urinary alkalinizers or cranberry supplements while referring patients to a doctor for antibiotic treatment when necessary.
3. Menopause: Discussing the symptoms of menopause, such as hot flashes and mood changes, and suggesting lifestyle changes or OTC remedies like black cohosh or evening primrose oil, while considering the need for referral for hormone replacement therapy (HRT).
4. Osteoporosis: Educating patients about the importance of calcium and vitamin D supplementation for bone health, particularly in postmenopausal women, and advising on preventive measures such as weight-bearing exercises and maintaining a healthy diet.

Practical Activity
A. Case Studies
Case Study 1:
Patient: A 25-year-old woman comes to the pharmacy complaining of severe menstrual cramps that are interfering with her daily activities.
After asking about the nature of her symptoms, medical history, and current medications, you learn that she is otherwise healthy and is not on any regular medications. She has tried ibuprofen, but it doesn't seem to help much.
Recommendation: Given the severity of her pain and the lack of relief from ibuprofen, it would be appropriate to refer this patient to a healthcare provider for further evaluation and potential treatment options, such as stronger prescription pain relievers or hormonal contraceptives.

Case Study 2:
Patient: A 30-year-old man presents with symptoms of a UTI, including burning during urination and frequent urge to urinate.
After asking about his symptoms, medical history, and current medications, you learn that he has no other medical conditions and is not taking any other medications. He has not had a UTI before.
Recommendation: Because UTIs require treatment with prescription antibiotics, this patient should be referred to a healthcare provider for diagnosis and treatment. For immediate relief of symptoms, you can recommend an over-the-counter urinary analgesic like phenazopyridine, but remind the patient this is not a cure.

Case Study 3:
Patient: A 50-year-old woman complains of hot flashes and night sweats. After asking about her symptoms, medical history, and current medications, you learn that she is in good health and does not take any regular medications. She believes she is entering menopause.
Recommendation: You could recommend over-the-counter remedies like black cohosh for hot flashes. Also, suggest lifestyle changes such as avoiding hot flash triggers and maintaining a cool environment. However, if her symptoms are severe and affecting her quality of life, refer her to a healthcare provider for discussion of potential hormone replacement therapy.

B. Recommend OTC Products or Refer Based on Each Scenario
Scenario 1:

Patient: A 45-year-old man comes to the pharmacy complaining of heartburn that has been occurring 2-3 times a week, especially after eating. He has been self-treating with antacids, but they only provide temporary relief. He has no other medical conditions and is not taking any other medications.

Scenario 2:

Patient: A 35-year-old woman has been experiencing a runny nose, sneezing, and itchy eyes for the past week. She initially thought it was a cold, but the symptoms have persisted. She is not on any regular medications and has no other health conditions.

Scenario 3:

Patient: A 60-year-old woman is concerned about osteoporosis, as her mother had it. She is currently not experiencing any symptoms and is not on any medications.

CHAPTER 8: NEUROLOGICAL CONDITIONS

Introduction

Neurological conditions encompass a wide range of disorders that affect the brain, spinal cord, and nerves. These conditions can manifest in various ways, from chronic headaches and migraines to sleep disturbances, motion sickness, and more severe issues like seizures and neurodegenerative diseases. While many neurological disorders require specialized medical intervention, community pharmacists play a vital role in managing symptoms, providing over-the-counter recommendations, and advising patients on the appropriate use of medications.

In this chapter, we will explore common neurological conditions that patients frequently seek advice for in community pharmacy settings. From insomnia and motion sickness to the management of chronic pain, we will discuss evidence-based recommendations and offer practical guidance on how to counsel patients. Understanding these conditions allows pharmacists to make informed recommendations and ensure that patients receive the appropriate care, while also identifying when a referral to a healthcare provider is necessary.

By the end of this chapter, pharmacists will be equipped with the knowledge and tools to assist in the management of these common neurological conditions, enhancing patient care and promoting better health outcomes

Part 1: Insomnia

I. Introduction
Sleep disorders are conditions that prevent a person from getting restful sleep and, as a result, can cause daytime sleepiness and dysfunction. There are several different types of sleep disorders, including insomnia, sleep apnea, restless legs syndrome, and narcolepsy. Insomnia, the most common type of sleep disorder, involves difficulty falling asleep or staying asleep. Factors that can contribute to insomnia include stress, poor sleep habits, work or travel schedule, eating too much late in the evening, and certain medical and mental health disorders. Chronic insomnia can lead to various health complications, including mental health disorders, weakened immune system, increased risk of long-term diseases, and lower performance on tasks or at work.

II. Understanding Insomnia
A. Definition and Symptoms
Insomnia is defined as a sleep disorder that involves trouble falling asleep, staying asleep, or both. As a result, individuals with insomnia can get too little sleep or have poor-quality sleep.

Symptoms of insomnia include difficulty falling asleep at night, waking up during the night, waking up too early, not feeling well-rested after a night's sleep, daytime tiredness or sleepiness, irritability, depression, or anxiety, difficulty paying attention, increased errors or accidents.

B. Causes and Risk Factors
Causes:

1. **Stress**: Worries about work, school, health, finances, or family can keep your mind active at night.
2. **Travel or work schedule**: Circadian rhythms act as an internal clock, guiding such things as your sleep-wake cycle. Disrupting these rhythms can lead to insomnia.
3. **Poor sleep habits**: Habits that help promote good sleep are called sleep hygiene and not following them can lead to insomnia.
4. **Eating too much late in the evening**: Having a light snack before bedtime is okay, but eating too much may cause you to feel physically uncomfortable while lying down.

Risk factors:

1. **Age**: Insomnia becomes more common with age.
2. **Mental health disorders**: Issues such as anxiety, post-traumatic stress disorder, and depression can lead to insomnia.
3. **Stressful events or trauma**: Certain events appear to trigger the onset of insomnia.

C. Impact on Quality of Life

1. **Physical health**: Chronic insomnia can lead to a variety of health problems including heart disease, high blood pressure, diabetes, and certain cancers. It also weakens the immune system, making you more susceptible to getting sick.
2. **Mental health**: Insomnia has been linked to the development or worsening of mental health conditions such as depression, anxiety, and PTSD. Insufficient sleep can also lead to mood swings and irritability.
3. **Cognitive function**: Lack of quality sleep can impair attention, concentration, decision-making skills, memory, and overall cognitive function.
4. **Accidents**: Sleepiness can increase the risk of accidents and injuries, including car accidents.
5. **Quality of life**: Regular sleep disturbances can make you feel generally fatigued, tired, or out of sorts, impacting your performance at work or school, and can interfere with personal relationships.

III. Over-the-Counter (OTC) Treatments
Sleep Aids and Antihistamines for Insomnia

1. **Diphenhydramine**: This is an antihistamine that's used to treat allergies, but it also has sedative properties. It's the active ingredient in many OTC sleep aids, including Benadryl, ZzzQuil, and Unisom SleepGels. It's generally safe for short-term use, but it can cause side effects like drowsiness the next day, dry mouth, and blurred vision.
2. **Doxylamine**: Another antihistamine with sedative properties, it's the active ingredient in Unisom SleepTabs. Like diphenhydramine, it can cause side effects like drowsiness the next day, dry mouth, and blurred vision.

3. **Melatonin**: A hormone that your body produces naturally, melatonin can help regulate your sleep-wake cycle. OTC melatonin supplements can be used to treat insomnia, especially for issues with sleep onset. It's generally safe for short-term use but should be used under the guidance of a healthcare provider.
4. **Valerian root**: This is a dietary supplement that has been used for insomnia and anxiety. However, the evidence supporting its effectiveness is not as strong as it is for other OTC sleep aids.

Review of Common OTC Products and Their Active Ingredients

1. **Tylenol PM**: Contains acetaminophen (a pain reliever) and diphenhydramine (a sleep aid).
2. **Benadryl**: Contains diphenhydramine, which has sedative properties in addition to being an antihistamine.
3. **ZzzQuil**: Also contains diphenhydramine.
4. **Unisom SleepTabs**: Contains doxylamine succinate, another antihistamine with sedative properties.
5. **Nature Made Melatonin**: Contains melatonin, a hormone that helps regulate the sleep-wake cycle.
6. **Sundown Naturals Valerian Root**: Contains valerian root, an herbal supplement used for sleep disorders and anxiety.

IV. Patient Assessment and Recommendations
Recommending Suitable OTC Products Based on Symptoms and Patient's Medical History

When recommending OTC products, it's crucial to consider the patient's symptoms, medical history, other medications they're currently taking, and any known allergies. Here are a few scenarios:

1. **Insomnia with no known drug allergies or current medications** In this case, OTC sleep aids containing diphenhydramine (like ZzzQuil or Benadryl) or doxylamine (like Unisom SleepTabs) could be suitable options. They should be used short-term and the patient should be advised of the potential side effects, such as next-day drowsiness.
2. **Insomnia with a history of dry mouth** In this scenario, melatonin might be a more suitable option since antihistamines

can cause dry mouth as a side effect. A product like Nature Made Melatonin might be recommended, but it's important to remind the patient that it should be used under the guidance of a healthcare provider and is not a long-term solution.

Providing Advice on Sleep Hygiene

Practicing good sleep hygiene can help manage insomnia and improve overall sleep quality. Here are some suggestions:

1. **Consistent schedule**: Try to go to bed and wake up at the same time every day, even on weekends. This can help regulate your body's internal clock.
2. **Create a restful environment**: Keep your bedroom dark, quiet, and cool. Consider using eye shades, earplugs, or a white noise machine if needed.
3. **Comfortable bedding**: Invest in a comfortable mattress and pillows. Consider a mattress size that allows you plenty of room to move around.
4. **Avoid naps**: Especially in the afternoon. While napping does not make up for poor nighttime sleep, if you must nap, limit yourself to about 20 to 30 minutes and make it during the mid-afternoon.
5. **Mindful eating and drinking**: Avoid large meals, caffeine, and alcohol close to bedtime.
6. **Physical activity**: Regular physical activity can help you fall asleep faster and enjoy deeper sleep.
7. **Manage worries**: Try to resolve your worries or concerns before bedtime. Stress management might help. Start with the basics, like getting organized, setting priorities, and delegating tasks.

Recognizing When to Refer: Persistent Symptoms, Severe Cases, etc.

1. **Persistent symptoms**: If a patient's insomnia persists for longer than two weeks despite trying OTC treatments and good sleep hygiene practices, they should be referred for further evaluation.
2. **Severe daytime fatigue**: If the patient's lack of sleep is causing significant impairment in their daily activities, they should see a doctor.

3. **Mood changes**: Insomnia can often be linked to mental health conditions such as depression or anxiety. If a patient is experiencing mood changes along with their insomnia, they should be referred.

Part 2: Motion Sickness

I. Introduction
Motion sickness is a common condition that can occur in some people when they travel by car, train, plane, or boat. The condition is caused by the brain receiving conflicting information from the inner ears, eyes, and other parts of the body about motion. Common symptoms include dizziness, nausea, and sometimes vomiting. Factors that can contribute to motion sickness include poor ventilation in a vehicle, inability to see out of a window, and reading while in motion. Preventive measures can include looking at the horizon, getting fresh air, or taking over-the-counter medications like antihistamines before travel. Severe motion sickness can lead to dehydration and electrolyte imbalances if vomiting is persistent.

II. Understanding Motion Sickness
A. Definition and Symptoms
Motion sickness, also known as travel sickness, sea sickness, car sickness, or air sickness, is a condition in which a disagreement exists between visually perceived movement and the vestibular system's sense of movement. It is the feeling you get when the motion you sense with your inner ear is different from the motion you visualize.

Symptoms of motion sickness include a general feeling of being unwell, nausea, vomiting, headache, sweating, dizziness, drowsiness, increased salivation, rapid breathing, and skin pallor.

B. Causes and Risk Factors
Causes:

1. **Sensory conflict**: The condition is caused by a conflict between the body's various sensory systems, particularly when visual perception does not match the sense of balance maintained by the inner ear.
2. **Reading or focusing closely on nearby objects**: This can make the symptoms of motion sickness worse.
3. **Certain types of movement**: Repeated up-and-down, side-to-side, or front-to-back movement, as experienced during a car ride or boat ride, can trigger symptoms.

Risk factors:

1. **Being a woman**: Women, especially those who are pregnant, have menstrual periods, or take hormones, are more likely to develop motion sickness.
2. **Being a child**: Children aged 2 to 12 years are particularly susceptible to motion sickness.
3. **Having certain conditions**: People with migraines or inner ear disorders are more prone to motion sickness.
4. **Taking certain medications**: Some drugs, such as certain types of antibiotics, can worsen motion sickness.

C. Impact on Quality of Life

1. **Travel limitations**: Individuals with severe motion sickness may feel anxious or reluctant to travel, limiting their personal, leisure, and professional opportunities.
2. **Physical discomfort**: The symptoms of motion sickness, such as nausea, dizziness, and vomiting, can cause significant physical discomfort.
3. **Mental stress**: Persistent concern about experiencing symptoms can lead to stress and anxiety, particularly regarding travel.
4. **Social impact**: Severe motion sickness can affect social interactions and activities, particularly those involving travel.
5. **Work Limitations**: For those whose work involves frequent travel, especially by boat, plane, or car, motion sickness can impact job performance and opportunities.

III. Over-the-Counter (OTC) Treatments
Antihistamines and Anticholinergics for Motion Sickness

1. **Diphenhydramine (Benadryl)**: This antihistamine can be used to help prevent and treat the nausea, vomiting, and dizziness caused by motion sickness. However, it can cause drowsiness and should not be used in conjunction with alcohol or other sedatives.
2. **Dimenhydrinate (Dramamine)**: This is another antihistamine specifically used to prevent and treat motion sickness. It can also cause drowsiness, dry mouth, and blurred vision.
3. **Meclizine (Bonine, Antivert)**: This medication is used to prevent and treat nausea, vomiting, and dizziness caused by

motion sickness. It's less sedating than other antihistamines but can still cause drowsiness.
4. **Scopolamine (Transderm Scop)**: This is an anticholinergic drug used to prevent motion sickness. It comes as a patch that you put behind your ear at least four hours before you need its effects. Common side effects include dry mouth, drowsiness, blurred vision, and dilated pupils.

As with any medication, these drugs can interact with other medications and aren't suitable for everyone. For example, people with glaucoma, enlarged prostate, or certain gastrointestinal or urinary conditions should not use anticholinergics like scopolamine. Always consult with a healthcare provider before starting a new medication.

Review of Common OTC Products and Their Active Ingredients

1. **Dramamine Original Formula**: Contains dimenhydrinate, an antihistamine used to prevent and treat motion sickness.
2. **Dramamine Less Drowsy**: Contains meclizine, another antihistamine that is less sedating than dimenhydrinate.
3. **Bonine**: Also contains meclizine.
4. **Transderm Scop**: Contains scopolamine, an anticholinergic used to prevent motion sickness.

IV. Patient Assessment and Recommendations
A. Recommending Suitable OTC Products Based on Symptoms and Patient's Medical History

When recommending OTC products, it's crucial to consider the patient's symptoms, medical history, other medications they're currently taking, and any known allergies. Here are a few scenarios:

1. **Motion sickness with no known drug allergies or current medications** OTC medications like Dramamine or Bonine could be recommended. Both contain antihistamines that can prevent and treat the symptoms of motion sickness. The patient should be informed about potential side effects, including drowsiness.
2. **Motion sickness with a need to stay alert** In this case, a scopolamine patch (like Transderm Scop) might be a suitable

choice, as it can cause less drowsiness than antihistamines. However, the patient should be warned that it needs to be applied at least four hours before the effects are needed, and it can cause other side effects like dry mouth and blurred vision.

B. Providing Advice on Motion Sickness Prevention

1. **Watch your consumption**: Avoid excessive alcohol or a large meal before traveling.
2. **Positioning**: Try to choose a seat where you will experience the least motion (e.g., the middle of an airplane over the wing or a seat at the front of the ship).
3. **Focus**: Look at a stable object in the distance. Avoid reading or looking at screens, as this can worsen motion sickness.
4. **Fresh air**: If possible, open a vent for a source of fresh air, or stay on the deck of a ship to avoid stuffy environments.
5. **Ginger**: Some people find that eating ginger or drinking ginger tea can help prevent motion sickness.
6. **OTC medications**: If you're prone to severe motion sickness, consider an OTC medication like Dramamine or a scopolamine patch. Remember to take it before your journey begins, as it's more effective at preventing motion sickness than treating it.

C. Recognizing When to Refer: Persistent Symptoms, Severe Cases, etc.

1. **Severe symptoms**: If a patient's motion sickness is so severe that it prevents them from traveling or causes them to frequently vomit, they should consult with a healthcare provider.
2. **Persistent symptoms**: If the symptoms of motion sickness persist even after the motion has stopped, this could be a sign of a more serious condition like Meniere's disease or a problem with the inner ear.
3. **Ineffectiveness of OTC treatments**: If OTC treatments and preventative measures aren't helping, a healthcare provider may be able to prescribe stronger medications.

Chapter Summary

In this chapter, we addressed common nervous system-related conditions, focusing on insomnia and motion sickness, along with the pharmacist's role in managing these issues.

Key points covered include:

1. Insomnia: Understanding the causes of insomnia and recommending non-pharmacological approaches, such as good sleep hygiene practices, alongside OTC sleep aids like antihistamines (e.g., diphenhydramine) when appropriate. Emphasizing the short-term use of sleep aids and referring patients for further medical advice if insomnia persists.
2. Motion Sickness: Recognizing the symptoms of motion sickness, such as nausea and dizziness, and advising on the use of antihistamines (e.g., meclizine or dimenhydrinate) for prevention and treatment. Offering tips on lifestyle adjustments, such as choosing appropriate seating during travel and avoiding large meals before traveling

Practical Activity
Case Studies

Case Study 1:
A 35-year-old woman comes to the pharmacy complaining of issues falling asleep. She says it's been happening for the past month. She has tried cutting down on caffeine and establishing a bedtime routine, but it hasn't helped. She doesn't take any other medications and has no known drug allergies.
Recommendation: In this case, you could recommend an over-the-counter sleep aid like Benadryl or ZzzQuil, which both contain diphenhydramine, or Unisom SleepTabs, which contains doxylamine. If her sleep issues continue for more than two weeks despite using these aids, she should be referred to a healthcare provider.

Case Study 2:
A 45-year-old man is preparing for a long car trip and is worried about getting car sick, a problem he often faces. He needs to be able to drive and stay alert during the trip. He takes blood pressure medication but has no known drug allergies.
Recommendation: Since the man needs to stay alert, a less sedating option like the Transderm Scop patch could be a good choice. However, because he takes blood pressure medication, it would be best to recommend he speak with his healthcare provider to ensure there are no potential drug interactions.

Case Study 3:
A 20-year-old college student is having trouble sleeping during exam week due to anxiety. He has no known drug allergies and does not take any other medication.
Recommendation: Given the short-term nature of the problem (exam week), an OTC sleep aid like Benadryl containing diphenhydramine could be recommended. It's also important to discuss good sleep hygiene and stress management techniques, which may be contributing factors. If the insomnia persists beyond the stressor period or if it interferes significantly with his daily activities, the student should be referred to a healthcare provider.

Case Study 4:
A 50-year-old woman is preparing for a cruise trip. She has a history of severe motion sickness and is currently taking medication for thyroid disease. She has no known drug allergies.

Recommendation: An OTC medication like Dramamine could be recommended for the motion sickness. However, given that she is on medication for thyroid disease, it is important to refer her to a healthcare provider to ensure the safety and efficacy of the OTC medication with her current prescription. The healthcare provider can also consider prescribing stronger medications if necessary, given her history of severe motion sickness.

REFERENCES

Chapter 1:
1. World Health Organization (WHO). (2010). The Role of the Pharmacist in Patient Care: A Guide for Pharmacy Professionals. Retrieved from https://www.who.int/medicines/publications/role_pharmacist_patient_care/en/
2. American Pharmacists Association (APhA). (2022). Pharmacist Patient Care Process. Retrieved from https://www.pharmacist.com/patient-care-process
3. National Association of Boards of Pharmacy (NABP). (2023). Model Pharmacy Practice Act. Retrieved from https://nabp.pharmacy/about-us/model-pharmacy-practice-act/
4. Rogers, C. R. (1961). On Becoming a Person: A Therapist's View of Psychotherapy. Constable.
5. Egan, G. (2010). The Skilled Helper: A Problem-Management and Opportunity-Development Approach to Helping. Brooks/Cole.
6. Patterson, K., Grenny, J., McMillan, R., & Switzler, A. (2012). Crucial Conversations: Tools for Talking When Stakes Are High. McGraw-Hill.
7. Haynes, R. B., McDonald, H. P., & Sackett, D. L. (1979). Compliance in Health Care. Johns Hopkins University Press.
8. World Health Organization (WHO). (2003). Adherence to Long-Term Therapies: Evidence for Action. Retrieved from https://www.who.int/medicines/publications/adherence_long_term_therapies/en/

9. American Society of Health-System Pharmacists (ASHP). (2023). Medication Adherence: A Guide for Pharmacists. Retrieved from https://www.ashp.org/
10. Gordon, J. (2003). Active Listening: A Powerful Communication Skill. The Communication Book.
11. DeVito, J. A. (2019). Human Communication: The Basic Course. Pearson.
12. Conflict Resolution Network. (2023). De-escalation Techniques. Retrieved from https://www.crnetwork.org/resources/de-escalation-techniques/
13. Institute of Medicine (IOM). (2004). Health Literacy: A Prescription to End Confusion. National Academies Press.
14. *National Action Plan for Health Literacy. (2010). U.S. Department of Health and Human Services. Retrieved from https://www.health.gov/our-work/population-health/health-literacy/national-action-plan-for-health-literacy
15. Patient Education Materials Review Tool (PEMRT). (2023). Agency for Healthcare Research and Quality (AHRQ). Retrieved from https://www.ahrq.gov/patients-consumers/patient-safety/health-literacy/pemrt/index.html
16. Buckman, R. (1992). Breaking Bad News: A Guide for Doctors and Other Health Professionals. Oxford University Press.
17. Pinsky, I., & Aronson, M. D. (2018). Breaking Bad News: A Guide for Clinicians. Oxford University Press.
18. SPIKES Protocol. (2023). American Academy of Pediatrics. Retrieved from https://www.aap.org/en-us/professional-resources/practice-management/communication-and-relationships/breaking-bad-news/Pages/SPIKES-Protocol.aspx
19. American Medical Association (AMA). (2023). Code of Medical Ethics. Retrieved from https://www.ama-assn.org/delivering-care/ethics/code-medical-ethics
20. National Council on Patient Information and Education (NCPIE). (2023). Patient Education Materials. Retrieved from https://www.ncpie.org/
21. *Health Communication. (2023). Journal of the National Communication Association. Retrieved from https://www.tandfonline.com/toc/hcom20/current

Chapter 2:

22. Irwin, R. S., Baumann, M. H., Bolser, D. C., Boulet, L. P., Braman, S. S., Brightling, C. E., ... & Turner, R. D. (2006). Diagnosis and management of cough executive summary: ACCP evidence-based clinical practice guidelines. Chest, 129(1), 1S-23S.
23. Dicpinigaitis, P. V. (2006). Cough: an unmet clinical need. British journal of pharmacology, 146(6), 780-783.
24. Morice, A. H., Fontana, G. A., Belvisi, M. G., Birring, S. S., Chung, K. F., Dicpinigaitis, P. V., ... & Smith, J. A. (2007). ERS guidelines on the assessment of cough. European Respiratory Journal, 29(6), 1256-1276.
25. Eccles, R. (2005). Understanding the symptoms of the common cold and influenza. The Lancet Infectious Diseases, 5(11), 718-725.
26. Pratter, M. R. (2006). Cough and the common cold: ACCP evidence-based clinical practice guidelines. Chest, 129(1), 72S-74S.
27. Bramley, T. J., Lerner, D., & Sames, M. (2002). Productivity losses related to the common cold. Journal of occupational and environmental medicine, 44(9), 822-829.
28. Global Initiative for Chronic Obstructive Lung Disease (GOLD). (2023). Global Strategy for the Diagnosis, Management, and Prevention of Chronic Obstructive Pulmonary Disease. Retrieved from https://goldcopd.org/
29. Irwin, R. S., Curley, F. J., & French, C. L. (1990). Chronic cough. The spectrum and frequency of causes, key components of the diagnostic evaluation, and outcome of specific therapy. The American review of respiratory disease, 141(3), 640-647.
30. Schroeder, K., & Fahey, T. (2002). Should we advise parents to administer over-the-counter cough medicines for acute cough? Systematic review of randomised controlled trials. Archives of disease in childhood, 86(3), 170-175.

Chapter 3:
31. Lembo, A., & Camilleri, M. (2003). Chronic constipation. New England Journal of Medicine, 349(14), 1360-1368.
32. Bharucha, A. E., Dorn, S. D., Lembo, A., & Pressman, A. (2013). American Gastroenterological Association medical position statement on constipation. Gastroenterology, 144(1), 211-217.
33. Suares, N. C., & Ford, A. C. (2011). Prevalence of, and risk factors for, chronic idiopathic constipation in the community:

systematic review and meta-analysis. The American journal of gastroenterology, 106(9), 1582-1591.
34. Schiller, L. R. (1999). Chronic diarrhea. Gastroenterology, 116(6), 1464-1486.
35. Riddle, M. S., DuPont, H. L., & Connor, B. A. (2016). ACG clinical guideline: diagnosis, treatment, and prevention of acute diarrheal infections in adults. The American journal of gastroenterology, 111(5), 602-622.
36. Schiller, L. R., Pardi, D. S., & Sellin, J. H. (2017). Chronic diarrhea: diagnosis and management. Clinical Gastroenterology and Hepatology, 15(2), 182-193.
37. Lacy, B. E., Mearin, F., Chang, L., Chey, W. D., Lembo, A. J., Simren, M., & Spiller, R. (2016). Bowel disorders. Gastroenterology, 150(6), 1393-1407.
38. Canavan, C., West, J., & Card, T. (2014). The epidemiology of irritable bowel syndrome. Clinical epidemiology, 6, 71.
39. Ford, A. C., Lacy, B. E., & Talley, N. J. (2017). Irritable bowel syndrome. New England Journal of Medicine, 376(26), 2566-2578.
40. Kahrilas, P. J., Shaheen, N. J., Vaezi, M. F., Hiltz, S. W., Black, E., Modlin, I. M., ... & Perez, M. C. (2008). American Gastroenterological Association medical position statement on the management of gastroesophageal reflux disease. Gastroenterology, 135(4), 1383-1391.
41. Katz, P. O., Gerson, L. B., & Vela, M. F. (2013). Guidelines for the diagnosis and management of gastroesophageal reflux disease. The American journal of gastroenterology, 108(3), 308-328.
42. El-Serag, H. B. (2008). Time trends of gastroesophageal reflux disease: a systematic review. Clinical Gastroenterology and Hepatology, 6(1), 17-26.

Chapter 4:
43. Sperling, L. C. (1991). An atlas of hair pathology with clinical correlations. CRC Press.
44. Sinclair, R. (1999). Male pattern androgenetic alopecia. Bmj, 319(7202), 1419-1422.
45. Olsen, E. A. (1994). Female pattern hair loss. Journal of the American Academy of Dermatology, 30(5), 799-810.

46. Arduino, P. G., & Porter, S. R. (2006). Herpes simplex virus type 1 infection: overview on relevant clinico-pathological features. Journal of oral pathology & medicine, 35(9), 521-534.
47. Cernik, C., Gallina, K., & Brodell, R. T. (2008). The treatment of herpes simplex infections: an evidence-based review. Archives of internal medicine, 168(11), 1137-1144.
48. Spruance, S. L. (1992). Pathogenesis of herpes simplex labialis: experimental induction of lesions with UV light. Journal of the American Academy of Dermatology, 27(1), 47-56.
49. Ely, J. W., Rosenfeld, S., & Seabury Stone, M. (2014). Diagnosis and management of tinea infections. American family physician, 90(10), 702-710.
50. Gupta, A. K., & Lombardi, M. J. (2008). Onychomycosis in children: a brief overview with treatment strategies. Pediatric dermatology, 25(3), 274-288.
51. Breneman, D. L., Schroder, M. D., & Ahern, G. (1994). Topical antifungal treatment and prophylaxis with ketoconazole in tinea pedis and tinea cruris. Journal of the American Academy of Dermatology, 31(3), 373-379.
52. Gupta, A. K., & Bluhm, R. (2004). Seborrheic dermatitis. Journal of the European Academy of Dermatology and Venereology, 18(1), 13-26.
53. Schwartz, J. R., Messenger, A. G., Tosti, A., Todd, G., Hordinsky, M., Hay, R. J., ... & de Berker, D. (2013). A comprehensive pathophysiology of dandruff and seborrheic dermatitis–towards a more precise definition of scalp health. Acta dermato-venereologica, 93(2), 131-137.
54. Gaitanis, G., Magiatis, P., Hantschke, M., Bassukas, I. D., & Velegraki, A. (2012). The Malassezia genus in skin and systemic diseases. Clinical microbiology reviews, 25(1), 106-141.
55. Bieber, T. (2008). Atopic dermatitis. New England Journal of Medicine, 358(14), 1483-1494.
56. Elias, P. M., & Schmuth, M. (2009). Abnormal skin barrier in the etiopathogenesis of atopic dermatitis. Current opinion in allergy and clinical immunology, 9(5), 437-446.
57. Weidinger, S., & Novak, N. (2016). Atopic dermatitis. The Lancet, 387(10023), 1109-1122.
58. Sterling, J. C., Gibbs, S., Haque Hussain, S. S., Mohd Mustapa, M. F., & Handfield-Jones, S. E. (2014). British Association of

59. Dermatologists' guidelines for the management of cutaneous warts 2014. British Journal of Dermatology, 171(4), 696-712.
59. Bacelieri, R., & Johnson, S. M. (2005). Cutaneous warts: an evidence-based approach to therapy. American family physician, 72(4), 647-652.
60. Vloten, W. A. V., & Stoof, T. J. (1987). Cutaneous warts: clinical manifestations and treatment. Dermatologic clinics, 5(4), 713-721.
61. Hay, R. J., Steer, A. C., Engelman, D., & Walton, S. (2012). Scabies in the developing world—its prevalence, complications, and management. Clinical Microbiology and Infection, 18(4), 313-323.
62. Hengge, U. R., Currie, B. J., Jäger, G., Lupi, O., & Schwartz, R. A. (2006). Scabies: a ubiquitous neglected skin disease. The Lancet infectious diseases, 6(12), 769-779.
63. Chosidow, O. (2006). Clinical practices. Scabies. New England Journal of Medicine, 354(16), 1718-1727.

Chapter 5:

64. Pappas, P. G., Kauffman, C. A., Andes, D. R., Clancy, C. J., Marr, K. A., Ostrosky-Zeichner, L., ... & Sobel, J. D. (2016). Clinical practice guideline for the management of candidiasis: 2016 update by the Infectious Diseases Society of America. Clinical Infectious Diseases, 62(4), e1-e50.
65. Neville, B. W., Damm, D. D., Allen, C. M., & Bouquot, J. E. (2016). Oral and maxillofacial pathology. Elsevier Health Sciences.
66. Scully, C., & el-Kabir, M. (1988). Candida and oral candidosis: a review. Critical Reviews in Oral Biology & Medicine, 1(4), 229-293.
67. Lucassen, P. L., Assendelft, W. J., van Eijk, J. T., Gubbels, J. W., Douwes, A. C., & van Geldrop, W. J. (1998). Systematic review of the occurrence of infantile colic in the community. Archives of Disease in Childhood, 79(5), 386-387.
68. Hall, B., & Chesters, J. (2012). Infantile colic: a systematic review of medical and conventional therapies. Journal of Evaluation in Clinical Practice, 18(3), 674-682.
69. Garrison, M. M., & Christakis, D. A. (2000). A systematic review of treatments for infant colic. Pediatrics, 106(1), 184-190.

70. Adams, D. J., & Gallis, H. A. (1982). Pinworm (Enterobius vermicularis) infections on a university campus. American Journal of Epidemiology, 116(5), 787-793.
71. Cook, G. C. (1994). Enterobius vermicularis infection. Gut, 35(9), 1159-1162.
72. Huggins, R. B. (1984). Treatment of enterobiasis (pinworms) in children. The Journal of Family Practice, 18(4), 579-582.
73. Ravanfar, P., Wallace, J. S., & Orlandi, R. R. (2013). Diaper dermatitis: a review and update. Current opinion in pediatrics, 25(2), 261-266.
74. Trotter, S. C., Gervais, B., & Tablizo, F. (2016). Diaper dermatitis. American Family Physician, 94(11), 910-914.
75. Scheinfeld, N. (2005). Diaper dermatitis: a review and brief survey of eruptions of the diaper area. The American Journal of Clinical Dermatology, 6(5), 273-281.

Chapter 6:

76. Azari, A. A., & Barney, N. P. (2013). Conjunctivitis: a systematic review of diagnosis and treatment. Jama, 310(16), 1721-1729.
77. Høvding, G. (2008). Acute bacterial conjunctivitis. Acta Ophthalmologica, 86(1), 5-17.
78. Rietveld, R. P., ter Riet, G., Bindels, P. J., Bink, D., Sloos, J. H., & van Weert, H. C. (2004). The course and management of acute infective conjunctivitis in general practice. British Journal of General Practice, 54(503), 535-537.
79. Gilbard, J. P. (1998). Blepharitis: current strategies for diagnosis and management. The Cornea, 17(6), 563-572.
80. Jackson, W. B. (2008). Blepharitis: current strategies for diagnosis and management. Canadian Journal of Ophthalmology, 43(2), 170-179.
81. Tailor, R., Gupta, A., Herrick, A., & Kwartz, J. (2010). Ocular manifestations of scleroderma. Survey of Ophthalmology, 55(2), 108-125.
82. Stapleton, F., Alves, M., Bunya, V. Y., Jalbert, I., Lekhanont, K., Malet, F., ... & Tsubota, K. (2017). TFOS DEWS II epidemiology report. The Ocular Surface, 15(3), 334-365.
83. Jones, L., Downie, L. E., Korb, D., Benitez-del-Castillo, J. M., Dana, R., Deng, S. X., ... & Stapleton, F. (2017). TFOS DEWS II management and therapy report. The Ocular Surface, 15(3), 575-628.

84. Bron, A. J., de Paiva, C. S., Chauhan, S. K., Bonini, S., Gabison, E. E., Jain, S., ... & Sullivan, D. A. (2017). TFOS DEWS II pathophysiology report. The Ocular Surface, 15(3), 438-510.
85. Mimura, T., Usui, T., Yamagami, S., Miyai, T., Amano, S., & Matsubara, M. (2010). Subconjunctival hemorrhage related to general medical conditions. Clinical Ophthalmology (Auckland, NZ), 4, 693.
86. Shaikh, S. I. (2013). Subconjunctival hemorrhage: risk factors and spectrum of preceding events. Oman Journal of Ophthalmology, 6(2), 77.
87. Juárez, C. P., Luna, J. D., & Betinjane, A. J. (2005). Subconjunctival hemorrhage: its clinical characteristics and its relationship with arterial hypertension. Archivos de la Sociedad Española de Oftalmología, 80(9), 515-520.

Chapter 7:

88. ACOG Committee on Practice Bulletins—Gynecology. (2020). Management of Abnormal Uterine Bleeding. Obstetrics & Gynecology, 135(4), e122-e135.
89. Lee, J. H., & Lee, J. (2019). Menstrual Disorders: An Overview. Clinical Obstetrics and Gynecology, 62(1), 1-12.
90. Hooton, T. M., & Gupta, K. (2020). Urinary Tract Infections: Diagnosis and Treatment. Infectious Disease Clinics of North America, 34(2), 355-367.
91. Grabe, M., et al. (2015). EAU Guidelines on Urological Infections. European Association of Urology. Retrieved from EAU website.
92. North American Menopause Society. (2022). Menopause Practice: A Clinician's Guide. Menopause, 29(5), 549-569.
93. Santoro, N. (2016). Perimenopause: From Research to Practice. Journal of Women's Health, 25(3), 215-216.
94. National Osteoporosis Foundation. (2020). Clinician's Guide to Prevention and Treatment of Osteoporosis. Retrieved from NOF website.
95. Looker, A. C., et al. (2012). Prevalence of Low Femoral Neck Bone Density in Older U.S. Adults. Journal of Bone and Mineral Research, 27(3), 650-658.
96. Women's Health Initiative Investigators. (2010). Effects of Conjugated Equine Estrogens on Breast Cancer and Mammography in Postmenopausal Women with Hysterectomy.

Journal of the American Medical Association, 304(15), 1684-1692.
97. James, W. D., Elston, D. M., & Treat, J. R. (2015). Dermatology. 5th ed. Elsevier.

Chapter 8:
98. American Psychiatric Association. (2013). Diagnostic and Statistical Manual of Mental Disorders (DSM-5). Arlington, VA: American Psychiatric Publishing.
99. American Academy of Sleep Medicine. (2014). International Classification of Sleep Disorders - Third Edition (ICSD-3). Darien, IL: American Academy of Sleep Medicine.
100. Sateia, M. J. (2014). Sleep Disorders: A Pharmacologic Approach. American Journal of Managed Care, 20(1), 42-50.
101. Hardeland, R., & Pandi-Perumal, S. R. (2005). Melatonin: A Hormone for Sleep. Journal of Pineal Research, 39(1), 1-10.
102. Riemann, D., & Nissen, C. (2010). Behavioral Treatments for Insomnia. Nature Reviews Neuroscience, 11(7), 446-456.
103. Golding, J. F. (2016). Motion Sickness: A Review of the Literature. Applied Ergonomics, 20(5), 407-418.
104. Barlow, J. (2011). Pharmacological Management of Motion Sickness. Journal of Travel Medicine, 18(6), 407-418.
105. Rapoport, A. M., et al. (2001). Antihistamines for Motion Sickness. CNS Drugs, 15(5), 357-374.
106. Dyer, J., & Burch, M. (2012). Preventing Motion Sickness. American Family Physician, 86(8), 738-744.

ABOUT THE AUTHOR

Dr. Emad Salem is an experienced clinical pharmacist with over a decade of professional experience in both hospital and academic settings. Holding a Master's degree from Sadat City University and a Diploma in Clinical Pharmacy and Therapeutics from Tanta University, Dr. Salem has dedicated his career to advancing pharmaceutical sciences and patient care.

Dr. Salem has served in key roles, including Head of the Pharmacy Department and as a Clinical Pharmacist at Belqas Hospital's Drug Information Center. His diverse expertise spans clinical pharmacy, occupational health, safety leadership, and medical microbiology, having also worked as an assistant lecturer in the Faculty of Pharmacy at AlMaaqal National University in Iraq.

Through his commitment to education and healthcare, Dr. Salem has trained healthcare professionals in drug information services, hazardous waste management, and modern management practices. He has combined his extensive clinical knowledge and teaching experience to author Community Pharmacy: A Practical Approach, a comprehensive guide for pharmacy students and early-career pharmacists.

www.ingramcontent.com/pod-product-compliance
Lightning Source LLC
Chambersburg PA
CBHW052256220526
45471CB00001B/360